THE BEST HEALTH
FLAVOURS

THE BEST HEALTH
FLAVOURS

Volume 2

Yusuf Wasiu

KJV
Scripture quotations marked KJV are from the Holy Bible, King James Version (Authorized Version). First published in 1611. Quoted from the KJV Classic Reference Bible, Copyright © 1983 by The Zondervan Corporation.

Any people depicted in stock imagery provided by Thinkstock are models, and such images are being used for illustrative purposes only.
Certain stock imagery © Thinkstock.

Print information available on the last page.

Rev. date: 05/30/2015

To order additional copies of this book, contact:
Xlibris
0-800-056-3182
www.xlibrispublishing.co.uk
orders@xlibrispublishing.co.uk
702208

CONTENTS

Introduction

You really need to know that, you are responsible for your health. Nobody will be happy, whenever he/she is sick. One cannot even really take care of himself/herself the way he/she does before the sickness. And if sickness is not put in check, it spreads rapidly from parents to their children, neighbours, and the whole city or country. Therefore, adequate health tips, and precautions, like washing our hands always, after using the toilet with soap and water thoroughly, is a very good health habit. Eating well prepared good food, also give the body adequate required energy and proteins, thus reducing the risks of fallen sick. Now, there is need to ask, why many women now have blocked fallopian tubes, without knowing? Now, fallopian tube is a major cause of female infertility. When there is blockage in the fallopian tube, it prevents spermatozoa from reaching an egg, to fertilize it. This leads to infertility. Many women still ovulate with blocked fallopian tube. It goes unnoticed a woman is trying to get pregnant. However, some women are born with blocked fallopian tubes. This is called congenital tubal obstruction. There are distal tubal occlusions, fimbrae issues, mid segment tubal obstructions

And proximal tubal occlusion. And the causes are, sexually transmitted infection, fibroids, ovarian cysts, endometriosis, ectopic pregnancy, pelvic inflammation disease, and miscarriage, or even abortion, where there were complications. A woman may experience certain symptoms, or nothing at all. Abdominal pain, fever, painful periods, strange looking, or smelling vaginal discharge, or feeling pains, while having sex, or passing urine. Also, fibroid is also called myoma. It affects two in five women. However, many women with myomas, do not experience any symptoms. It affects mostly people of child bearing age. Uterine fibroids may leads to some complications durings pregnancy, such as, bleeding during first trimester, placenta displacement. Increased estrogen may cause accelerated fibroid growth. If the fibroid grows during pregnancy, then there is a risk that it will move or tear the placenta. A caeserian birth will be necessary, when multiple fibroids located in the lower part of the uterus block the birth canal. Premature labour may set in. Miscarriage do prevent the embryo or foetus from developing, and ultimately cause a miscarriage. Generally, myomas are not removed during pregnancy, due to the increased risk of haemorrhage. It is possible, that between week 12 - 22, the blood supply to the fibroid may stop, causing it to turn red, and die. When this occur, it causes intence abdominal pains, and contractions, which may lead to premature labour, or even miscarriage. In spite of the various complications, many women with myoma, who do get pregnant, have normal pregnancies, and successful deliveries. However, the effect during pregnancy is unpleasant. The best is to get rid of fibroid before pregnancy. Moreover, it render many women infertile. The symptoms of uterine fibroid are, heavy, and prolonged bleeding, pelvic pain, or pressure, pain in the back of the legs, pressure on the bladder, pressure on the bowel, lower bacl pain, and pain during sexual intercourse. While a number of medical treatment exists for fibroid, but they come with risk and negative side effects. It is an external object, that grows in the womb, which is not suppose to be there. You now see few reasons, why you should take health and wellness tips, and informations serious. Well, the ball is in our court. We all are the architects of our good health and wellness.

Sickness is a Spirit

Every perfect gift comes from God. Behind every sickness is Satan James 4:7. Resist the devil and he will flee. Luke 13:11-12 "Woman thou art loose from your infirmity i.e sickness. Mark 9:25. "Deaf and dump spirit come out of her". Until you deal with Satan, you can not enjoy freedom. Resist the devil. There are spirits behind every sickness. Please handover everything to the Lord.

Sickness is of the devil, the world had sold lie to us. Stand on the Word of God. Mark 5:8-11 "And he said to him, come out of the man, you unclean spirit". The man was made whole.

Laugh Your Way to Good Health.

Police: A pastor was driving on the express way, when he met a team of mobile police men (other wise known as mopol in Nigeria), who quite naturally, wanted something from him. Since he was not prepared to play their games, they asked for his papers, and having combed, through everything without, any offence with which to nail the "stubborn" pastor, they now asked him to open the bonnet of his car. A careful scrutiny of the engine number against what was on paper revealed that the letter 'U' was an written in such a way that it can be mistaken for letter 'V'. That was all the officer-in-charge needed to shout "stolen vehicle"! Sensing trouble, even when he knew he committed no offence, the pastor called the officer in-charge, to say he was a priest, to which the officer, replied. "Please if you are indeed a pastor, then you must have a bible in your car, right, bring it," the pastor did as was commanded after which the officer now ordered:" "Please read Matthew 5:25 and 26 to me." The incredulous pastor opened to the recommended passage and read: "Settle matters quickly with your adversary who is taking you to court. Do it while you are still with him on the way, or he may hand you over to a judge, and the judge may hand you over to the officer, and you may be thrown into prison. I tell you the truth; you will not get out until you have paid the last penny."

Comment: What!!! This is true!!! Funny how even villains can use the bible to justify their evil deeds.

The Oldest Profession

A physician, an engineer, and attorney were discussing who among them belonged to the oldest of the three professions represented. The physician said," remember, on the sixth day, God took a rib from Adam and fashioned Eve, making him the first surgeon. Therefore, medicine is the oldest profession.

The engineer replied, "But before that, God created the heavens, and earth, from chaos, and confusion. Therefore engineering is an older profession than medicine."

Then the lawyer spoke up, "Yes" he said, "But who do you think created all of the chaos and confusion?

Never take alcohol, it is poisonous like snake's venom. Alcohol destroys the liver and causes liver cirhosis in the body. Such liver would not be able to perform myriad of its functions effectively anymore, thus causing early painful death.

A guy goes into a bar, in America, and asks, for three separate shots of whiskey, he drinks one, wait a little bit, then drinks the second one, wait a little bit, then more, then and then drinks the third one. This goes on for a few days, and finally, the bar tender tells him: "You know sir, I can put all the three shots in one glass for you." The guy replied. "No, I prefer, it this way. You see, I'm very close to my two brothers. They are both in abroad, and this represents, a drink for each of us. When I drink like this, I feel like we are drinking together again, all three of us."

This goes on for several months, and then one day, the guy walk into the pub, and ask for only two shots. The bartender is worried that maybe something happened to one of his brothers. "Is everything o.k.?" He asks.

"What do you mean," answers the guy. "Well, for months you have been asking for three shots. Now you order two. Did something happen to one of your brothers?

The bartender asks. "No," replies, the guy, "they're fine. It's just that I quit drinking".

Professor and Fisherman

A professor boarded a canoe from one side of the river bank, with a fisherman, that paddle the canoe. The professor asked the fisherman if he know about geography? The fisher man said no, he also asked him if he know about geophysics and algebra, while the fisherman equally replied no. The professor now said that, the fisher man was disadvantaged, also that he is a dullard.

But while in the middle of the river, the canoe was about to capsize due to heavy wind that was blowing. The fisherman now asked the professor if he can swim? The professor replied, No. The fisherman now told him, "You just lost your life" he jumped into the river and started swimming to the river bank.

Zebra Cross

A hunter travels to Lagos for the first time from village. He was about to cross the road, when a law enforcement agent (Federal Road Safety Corps member) now directed him to use the zebra cross, on reaching his destination. He thought about the zebra that was crossing the road, and thought of killing it. He loaded his gun, and came to the zebra crossing point at night to wait for the zebra, so as to kill it. The following morning, no zebra crossed, except human beings. He was now asked, why is he with the gun. He told them, he want to kill the zebra that they say always cross the road here!

White Man and Balloons

A white man with blue blood was standing beside a fountain in a park, in New Jersey, and was blowing air into balloons of different colours, and releasing them in to the sky.

A black boy walked up to him, and asked "Will the black balloon also fly in the sky as the other balloon, if air is blowing inside it"? The white man replied yes, and picked the black balloon and blew air in it, and release it to the sky. Off it went up, like the other balloons, the white man now said "It's not the colour that matters, but it is the air inside" "Now a black man is even the American president!

Pastor and God (Listen to God)

A young pastor died, 25 years old married, with two kids. His friend a pastor too was very angry with God, for allowing his friend to die, he was asking God why? Why?

The day of burial came and every member of their church and friends went to the cemetery to bury the dead pastor. The dead pastor's, friend still continue to blame and ask God why did he allow his friend to die? God did not say anything. After the burial, every body went home. The dead pastor's friend was driving himself alone in the car on the high way, when he heard a voice telling him to stop and park the car! He neglected the voice and continued to drive on, at a point, he still heard the voice telling him to stop and park the car. He also ignored God's instruction the second time.

The third time, God told him loudly to stop, and park the car. The pastor now thought somebody was hiding in his back seat, and stopped and parked the car, he was about to open his door at the driver side, to come down to look properly for the person, when a 40 foot trailer container moving on top of bridge across the express on top, of the road, and was loaded with heavy machines fell off the bridge after loosing control, just about twelve feet in front of his car.

God now told him that, his friend died, because he did not listen to His instruction, and the same thing almost happen to him too, he should be warned and always adhere to His instructions.

Arthritis

Arthritis is a disease that causes pain and loss of movement of the joints. The word arthritis literally means joint inflammation (arth = joint, ritis = inflammation), and refers to more than 100 different diseases.

Arthritis can be very painful condition, but there are many natural therapies that can help in both arthritis management and prevention. Examples are (a) homoephaty for arthritis, (b) herbal therapies for arthritis (c) using diet and supplements to help arthritis, the role of exercise and physical therapy in arthritis treatments and prevention. (c) other treatments to manage or prevent arthritis.

Arthritis affects the movements you rely on for everyday activities. Arthritis is usually chronic. This means that it can last on and off for a life time. There are over 100 kinds of arthritis that can affect many different areas of the body. In addition to the joints, some forms of arthritis are associated with diseases of other tissues and organs in the body. People of all ages, including children and young adults can develop arthritis.

Normally, inflammation is the way the body responds to an injury or to the presence of disease agents, such as viruses or bacteria. During this reaction, many cells of the body's defense system (called the immune system) rush to the injured area to wipe out the cause of the problem, clean up damaged cells and repair tissues that have been hurt. Once the "battle" is won, the inflammation normally goes away and the area becomes healthy again.

In many forms of arthritis, the inflammation does not go away as it should. Instead, it becomes part of the problem, damaging healthy tissues of the body. This may result in more inflammation and more damage - continuing cycle. The damage that occurs can change the bones and other tissues of the joints, sometimes affecting their shape and making movement hard and painful. Diseases in which the immune system malfunctions and attacks healthy parts of the body are called auto immune diseases.

Rheumatoid arthritis: Arthritis pain and inflammation of joints has many forms. Rheumatoid arthritis can be one of the most disabling types of arthritis. Its cause varies, from a few symptoms to severe and painful deformities. Three times as many women as men are affected, usually at a fairly young age (between 25 and 50years). The disease may come on slowly or appear suddenly.

Rheumatoid Arthritis typically affects the small finger joints, wrists, knees and toes. All joints of the body, however, are potential targets. Along with swelling and pain of joints, some of the early symptoms of the disease may include fatigue, loss of appetite, weight loss and fever. Stiffness in the joints and surrounding muscles that lasts for several hours after getting up in the morning is a regular symptom. Some times the disease involves other organs, causing damage to the heart, lungs, eyes, skin and nerves.

Many individuals with rheumatoid arthritis feel their arthritis is influenced by the weather, stress, temperature and exercise. A few have periods of remission when the disease seems to have gone away. Unfortunately, in most cases, the symptoms eventually return. The cause of rheumatoid arthritis is unknown. Some scientists feel that it may result from an infection, but there is no evidence that it is contagious. For whatever reason, the joint lining becomes very inflamed and thickened, slowly destroying cartilage and bone. The goal of treatment is to halt the inflammation and prevent the destruction of joints. Medical supervision is a must, because, this form of arthritis can be crippling, other organs may be affected and all treatment may, on occasion, cause side effects.

Doctors now have many ways of treating rheumatoid arthritis. Large doses of aspirin or aspirin - like drugs can be effective in reducing pain and inflammation. If the arthritis is aggressive, drugs called DMARDS or SAARDS (Disease-Modifying Anti-Rheumatic

Drugs, or Slow-Acting Anti-Rheumatic Drugs) such as anti-malarial may be used. Certain immuno suppressants biologic response modifiers corticosteroids, or gold therapy may be used. All these drugs require close supervision, since they may have hazardous side effects. Rest, heat, and physical therapy are important adjuncts to drug therapy. A healthy diet and exercise also helps patients retain mobility and strength, maintaining a positive attitude although, there is no scientific evidence that eating or not eating certain foods reduces or aggravates symptoms of rheumatoid arthritis. Omega-3 fatty acids (found in certain fish and plant seed oils) may reduce the inflammation of rheumatoid arthritis.

Joint deformity or pain is some times so severe that surgery is the best alternative. A patient can have added years of mobility due to the hip, elbow, shoulder, and knee replacements that can be performed today. Surgeries include joint replacement (replacing the joint with an artificial joint). Tendons reconstruction (reconstructing damaged tendons) and synovectomy (removal of the inflamed tissue). The use of a splint or brace can also help straighten some joints. Although surgery cannot cure all deformities, advances in the field have given rheumatoid patients, who previously would have been wheelchair-bound, the ability to continue in relatively normal lives. One form of chronic arthritis (less widely known) is one that attacks children.

Juvenile rheumatoid arthritis. This may start with symptoms as general fever and rash, and it may take a long time for a definite diagnosis to be reached. Some children complain of swelling and stiffness in a few scattered joints. When the disease threatens the function of the joints, skilled professional treatment is called for to prevent permanent deformity. The disease in its juvenile form often stops progressing within 10 years, but the damage may be permanent and cause further deterioration of the joints. The major concern for the child, parent and doctor is to provide treatment that will spare the child a deformity that might persist long after the disease itself has disappeared.

Osteoarthritis - is a disease that causes the breakdown of joint tissue, leading to joint pain and stiffness. It can affect any joint, but commonly occurs in the hips, knees, feet and spine. It also may affect some finger joints, the joint at the base of the thumb and the joint at the base of the big toe. It rarely affects the wrists, elbows, shoulders, ankle or jaw, except as a result of injury or unusual stress. Osteoarthritis is one of the oldest and most common diseases in humans. It probably affects almost every person over age 60 to some degree, but only some have it badly enough to notice any symptoms. Osteoarthritis is also known by many other names, such as degenerative joint disease, arthrosis, osteo arthrosis, or hypertrophic arthritis.

Treatment of Arthritis

Treatments for arthritis include rest and relaxation, exercise, proper diet, medication, and instruction about the proper use of joints and ways to conserve energy. Other treatments include the use of pain relief methods and assistive devices, such as splints or braces. In severe cases, surgery may be necessary. The doctor and the patient work together to develop a treatment plan that helps the patient maintain or improve his or her life style. Treatment plans usually combine several types of treatment and vary depending on the rheumatic condition and the patient.

a. **Homoephaty for Arthritis**

Homoephaty is a system of remedies, that are based on the belief that, tiny amounts of natural substances can be used to stimulate the body's own defenses, against a disease, in this case, arthritis. The whole body is taken into account. Some common, homeophatic remedies include arsenicum albub, calcarea carbonica, pulsatilla, and rhus toxicodemdron.

b. **Herbal therapies for arthritis**

There are many herbal therapies, that can be useful in the treatment of arthritis. Devil's claw is an anti-inflammatory, and can act as a pain killer. Boswella Serrapa is capable of decreasing inflammatory pathways, stopping cartilage breakdown, and increasing blood supply to the joints. Other herbs that can help include nettle leaf and ginger.

c. Using diet and supplements to help arthritis.

If you suffer from any form of arthritis, it is important to follow a healthy diet, and to introduce certain supplements. People with arthritis may be deficient in B vitamins, vitamin C, vitamin E, and beta carotene. Ensure that your diet is rich in vitamin E, and the anti-oxidants lutein and lycopene. Eat diet that is rich in all of the above vitamins in order to help prevent the onset of arthritis as well as reducing pain if you already suffer from it. Omega three oils are also helpful. These dietary fatty acids, regulate inflammation in the body, and they are capable of reducing the chronic inflammation associated with arthritis - eating foods rich in omega – three, and taking a daily supplement, can reduce your dependence on anti-inflammatory medications, or may even eliminates the need to take them altogether.

There are several supplements that may be extremely beneficial. Perhaps the most important of these is glucosamine sulphate. Glucosamine is a naturally occuring substance in the body, that is used to make, cartillage but as we grow older, the body produces less of it, requiring supplementation. Glucosamine stimulates the repair of cartilage in the body and thus reduces pain. Chondroitin sulphate is another supplement that may be of use. Chondroitin is abundant within the cartilage and is responsible for attracting and holding water within the cartilage-MSM. Organic sulphur is a natural way to reduce inflammation in joints, and supports healing, by increasing blood flow, and delivering nutrients to the injured areas.

Medications

A variety of medications are used to treat rheumatic diseases. The type of medication depends on the rheumatic disease and on the individual patient. At this time, the medications used to treat most rheumatic diseases do not provide a cure, but rather limit the symptoms of the disease. The one exception is treatments for infections arthritis. If caught early enough, arthritis associated with an infection (such as Lyme disease) can usually be cured with antibiotics. The doctor may delay using medications, until a definite diagnosis is made, because medications can hide important symptoms (such as fever and swelling), and thereby interfere with diagnosis. Patients taking any medication, either prescription or over-the-counter, should always follow the doctor's instructions. The doctor should be notified immediately if the medicine is making the symptoms, worse or causing other problems such as an upset stomach, nausea, or headache. The doctor may be able to change the dosage or medicine to reduce these side effects.

Analgesics (pain relievers) such as aspirin and other Nonsteroidal Anti-Inflammatory Drugs (NSAIDs) such as ibuprofen and acetaminophen are used to reduce the pain caused by many rheumatic conditions. Aspirin and other NSAIDs have the added benefit of decreasing the inflammation associated with arthritis.

Aspirin and other NSAIDs can have side effects, such as stomach irritation, that can be reduced by changing the dosage or the medication. The dosage will vary depending on the particular illness and the overall health of the patient. The doctor and patient must work together to determine which analgesic to use and the appropriate amount. If analgesics do not ease the pain, the doctor may use other medications, depending, on the diagnosis.

Corticosteroids, such as prednisone, cortisone, solymedrol solumedrol, and hydrocortisone, are used to treat many rheumatic conditions because they decrease inflammation and suppress the immune system. The dosage of these medications will vary, depending on the diagnosis and the patient again, the patient and doctor must work together to determine what dose is best for the patient. Side effects may occur after long-term of use of corticosteroids. These include stretch marks, excessive hair growth, osteoporosis, high blood pressure, damage to the arteries, high blood sugar, infections, and cataracts.

d. Rest, exercise, diet, and physical therapy in arthritis treatment and prevention.

People who have a rheumatic disease such as arthritis should develop a comfortable balance between rest and activity. One sign of many rheumatic conditions is fatigue. Patients must pay attention to signals from their bodies. For example, when experiencing pain or fatigue, it is important to take a break and rest. Too much rest, however, may cause muscles and joints to become stiff.

Physical exercise can reduce joint pain and stiffness and increase flexibility, muscle strength, and endurance. It also helps with weight reduction, and contributes to an improved sense of well-being. Before starting any exercise program, people with arthritis should talk with their doctor. Regular exercise can help to prevent arthritis and also improve itself. If you already suffer from joint pain, you may find that resistance exercise is helpful. The key is to do moderate exercise, and try not to put too much impact on to your joints. Walking, swimming, and yoga are just three beneficial forms of exercise. Combining exercise with physical therapy may reduce pain, stop the arthritis, from getting worse, and even prevent, or delay the necessity of a joint replacement.

Another important part of a treatment program is a well-balanced diet. Along with exercise, a well balanced diet helps people manage their body weight and stay healthy. Weight control is important to people who have arthritis because extra weight puts extra pressure on some joints, and can aggravate many types of arthritis.

Regular exercise can help to prevent arthritis and also improve the condition after it has established itself. If you already suffer from joint pain, you may find that resistance exercise is helpful. The key is to do moderate exercise, and try not to put too much impact onto your joints. Walking, swimming, and yoga are just three beneficial forms of exercise. Combining exercise with physical therapy may reduce pain, stop the arthritis, from getting worse, and even prevent, or delay the necessity of a joint replacement.

Heat and Cold Therapies

a. **Heat and cold** can both be used to reduce the pain, and inflammation of arthritis. Both therapies come in different forms, and the patient and doctor can determine which form works best. Heat and cold therapies, are equally effective, in reducing pain, although they are usually avoided in acute gout. Heat therapy increases blood flow, tolerance for pain, and flexibility. Heat therapy can involve treatment with paraffin wax, microwaves, ultrasound, or moist heat. Physical therapists are needed to apply paraffin wax, or use microwave or ultra sound therapy, but patients can apply moist heat themselves. Some ways to apply moist heat include placing warm towels or hot packs on the inflamed joint or taking a warm bath or shower.

b. **Cold therapy** numbs the nerves around the joint (which reduces pains), and relieves inflammation and muscle spasms. Cold therapy can involve cold packs, ice massage, soaking in cold water, or over-the-counter sprays and ointments that cool the skin and joints.

Hydro Therapy, Mobilization Therapy, and Relaxation Therapy.

a. **Hydrotherapy**, involves exercising or relaxing in warm water, which helps relax tense muscles and relieve pain. Exercising in a large pool is easier because water takes some weight off painful joints. This type of exercise improves muscle strength and joint movement.

b. **Mobilization therapies** include traction (gentle, steady pulling), massage, and manipulation (using the hands to restore normal movement to stiff joints). When done by a trained professional, these methods can help control pain, increase joint motion, and improve muscle and tendon flexibility.

c. **Relaxation therapy** helps reduce pain by teaching people various ways to release muscle tension throughout the body. In one method of relaxation therapy, known as progressive relaxation, the patient tightens a muscle group and then slowly releases the tension. Doctors and physical therapists can teach patients progressive relaxation and other relaxation techniques.

Assistive Devices:

The most common assistive devices for treating arthritis pain are splint and braces, which are used to support weakened joints or allow them to rest. Some of these devices prevent the joint from moving;

others allow some movement. A splint or brace should be used only when recommended by a doctor or therapist, who will show the patient the correct way to put the device on, ensure that it fits properly, and explain when and for how long it should be worn. The incorrect use of a splint or brace can cause joint damage, stiffness and pain.

Surgery

Surgery may be required to repair damage to a joint after trauma (a torn meniscus, for example) or to restore function or relieve pain in a joint damaged by arthritis. The doctor might recommend arthroscopic surgery, bone fusion, (surgery in which bones in the joint are fused or joined together), or arthroplasty (also known as total joint replacement, in which the damaged joint is removed and replaced with an artificial one).

Other Treatment to Manage or Prevent Arthritis

There are many other treatments that can help in the management, of arthritis. Here is a brief overview of just some of them.

a. **Massage:** This is beneficial as it increases flexibility and mobility. It also decreases pain and inflammation, relieves aches and stiffness and promotes a feeling of overall relaxation.

b. **Acupuncture** helps to stimulate the energy flow and can also help the body to release pain-relieving chemicals. This equals less pain.

c. **The Alexander technique** analyses whole body patterns and teaches an improved stance, so that people are able to stand and move efficiently. By moving in a better way, we eliminate tension which may be responsible for many, ailments including arthritis.

d. **Aromatherapy:** This involves the use of oils from flowers, plants, and trees, in combination with massage, baths or steam inhalation. By using the right mixture of essential oils, it may help with relaxation, pain relief, and decreasing, tiredness.

e. **Chiropractic** has been used for a long time in relieving arthritis. By adjusting the joints of the spine and the limbs, mobility will be increased, and the body will be relieved of tension, and stress.

f. **Osteopathy:** This involves the manipulation of the body in order to restore normal action and decrease pain. It is good for improving mobility, but it should not be used by those that have inflamed joints or osteoporosis.

g. **Reflexology:** This involves massaging the feet, and palms of the hand to improve the rest of the body. It is excellent for stress management, and overall health maintenance. **Osteoporosis, disease of the bones, causes bone fracture in women.**

Bones don't heal themselves with a sticking plaster, osteoporosis is a disease suffered by old ladies, and women should be encourage to consider their bone health before it is too late.

Treatment: The most common treatment for osteoporosis is biphosphonates – drugs, that slow down the rate at which old bone is absorbed, and help the cells, that make new bone work more efficiently. These are normally taken as a daily, weekly, or monthly pill. But to be effective, the medication does need to be taken regularly and at specific times of the day - generally an hour before food, which can become problematic. Indeed, there are many women who neglect taking their medication.

Seventy per cent didn't take it regularly - almost half of them deliberately, because of the fear of side-effects, such as irritation to the gut, or because they were confused by the instructions. The good news is that generally, it is never too late for properly taken medication to make a difference. You are not going to be able to get the bones back to the way they used to be, but you can retain their strength and stop them from getting worse. A patient because of her blind spot in regular taking of the pills, was advised to be taking a once-a-year treatment. Zoledronic acid, a form of biphosphonate, is given during an annual 15 minutes infusion. It can reduce the risk of a hip fracture, by more than 40 per cent, and a spinal fracture by more than 70 per cent. Although available in Britain, it's more expensive than other treatments and is generally given only to those for whom other medication, have not worked, or who've had side-effects.

People should discuss with their doctor, if they do not think they are on the right medication. Generally, they will be started on the cheapest, which might not be the right drug for them. The problem we have is that there is a lack of awareness among people, about osteoporosis. They will never think about the health of the bone until a fracture has occurred. The earlier, the disease can be caught, the better, as medication can reduce the risk of a fracture by as much as 70 per cent. The world health organization has introduced a questionnaire called the FRAX system, which peoples can use to assess the risk of fracturing a bone due to osteoporosis. However, it is not yet, mandatory. It's estimated that without changes to the diagnostic system, the number of fracture caused by osteoporosis will double in 60 years.

A patient said "I think it's strange that women get told to have a mammogram regularly to check their breasts, for cancer, but are not urged to get their bones checked for osteoporosis.

Tragically, many people, break bones, and are then bed-ridden for a long time because they did not know they had the disease. Getting older brings lot of strange surprises. It affects your body in ways you don't expect.

How Couple Can Cope With Infertility

Couples facing infertility are advised to be open-minded as possible. To cope with infertility, it is quite necessary to open the lines of communication as often as possible. Developing the essential communication skills can help strengthen a couple's connection with each and with other people.

a. **Both husband and wife must share the problem.** The first thing every infertile couple should accept, is that, no matter which partner (the man or woman) is identified as having the problem. It is something that should be shared by both of them. Another point to note is that in addition to the ability to work through all issues related to infertility, the ability to communicate in a helpful and clear way is just important to getting through the process. Simple thing, like sitting down to, and having a deep, serious conversation that generate thought provoking issues may not be as easy as it sounds, probably because the concerned individuals, allow themselves to be forced to focus on the pain, and stress of their situation. Since it can be depressing when conversation outlines series of depressing issues, infertile couples often avoid conversation about infertility. Effective communication techniques abound that men and women can develop during their struggles with infertility. For instance, taking time to talk about the problem rather than putting blame on the other person works better. It helps make the commitment to talk to each other. When fertility is the issue, each person needs to understand and appreciate the other's feelings and desires. It is not a matter of "tolerating" the other person's feelings or desires. It is more important to make them a part of sharing a difficult joint project together. The couple needs to be a team.

b. **Husband and wife need to talk to one another!** Finding something good to talk about is essential. Some times, in the midst of infertility treatment, it might be hard to come up with a positive topic, but it does not have to be a complicated matter.

An item heard on the radio, read on the internet, a conversation with a colleague at work, or something funny that happened during the day might make positive topics. This helps relieve some of the pressure that you and your partner are facing. If the communication process deteriorates, to the point, that either partner is seeking understanding from others outside of the relationships. It could become the trigger for bigger problems in the future. When I say there should be more communication. I am talking of a positive communication. If either or both persons don't feel like their needs are being met, and the other person does not understand them, then more communication can be negative. There are various other ways in which men and women approach communication. On their own part, women have a need to process things, and to sometimes talk about things at greater lengths, than men, who may be more focused, on finding out how to fix the problem, and may not want to focus on other activities that might distract both partners; activities like reading a book, or story about infertility, cleaning up the dishes, or watching television might be a lot easier than having a face-to-face conversation. But I would rather insist that it would do more good for the relationship of an infertile couple to focus on the issue.

Taking active part in support group activities can be a productive coping mechanism. Couples can come together and there is a real normalizing of the experience, where women realize they're not the only one who feel the way they do, and men hear that their wives aren't crazy, and that other women are going through this and they also get support for themselves. It is also not out of place for the support group, to plan weekend retreats, for couples facing this challenge.

c. **Husband and wife should listen actively:** Active listening is an effective technique that can be used during communication. Sometimes, the balance gets lost when one partner is doing most of the talking. It may sound awkward at first, but trying, to balance the amount of time each person talks and listens helps tremendously. Using a timer to do this at first might be a helpful tool. What is important is to listen "actively." Techniques like leaning towards, the person speaking, nodding during conversation, or making eye contact with the other person as he or she is speaking can help communicate with the other person, what you thought you heard him or her say in your known words. Sometimes, it helps to repeat it word for word. However, it should be kept in mind that active listening is not problem-solving, but simply a means to clarify what the other person has said as a way to promote understanding in relationships. It may also be an effective technique to take turns addressing each partner's needs in a series of conversations. Making time to listen to the needs of one partner over another, one at a time, is important.

d. **Husband versus wife:** When women feel distraught or anxious about infertility, issue they are facing, they may want to talk about them at length, but this may be overwhelming for their partners, who may decide to close themselves, off to communication even before it starts, making women feel more isolated and alone. What can help in this situation is for couples to decide that they will talk about the problem, but only for a fixed period of time. Let's say 20 minutes everyday. At the end of 20 minutes, they'll be finished, with it, and can move onto other things. It is important to be able to talk about the infertility experience while going through it. It is also important not to make it the only thing that is talked about.

e. **Husband and wife must take responsibility:** Expressing yourself during communication helps. Using statements beginning with "I" is an essential tool. These "I" statements should be as simple and concise as possible to allow the other person respond in an uncomplicated a statement may be, the higher the odds that misinterpretation will result. "I" statements express exactly how one feels about the situation without blaming the other person. The speaker essentially takes responsibility for his or her own thoughts feelings without requiring anything from the other person. This way, words are not being put into anybody's mouth, and assumptions are avoided. Like I said earlier, different couples have different coping styles, so this is not to suggest that couples all of a sudden start trying to adopt a system of communicating they have not had in building a close relationship. If you feel good about your system, no matter how bad it may look to others, and you are happy with your relations, go on with what you've got. Any kind of communication is harder during stress, but if you have a super-ordinate goal that you share, it will go a long way towards carrying you through the tough times.

f. **Some essential tips for communicating with friends and family:** Knowing how much detail you and your partner are readily ready to share with family or friends and as much as possible, respect each other's need for privacy about specific details.

– It helps to rehearse exactly what to say. Specific words like the use of "infertility" or "we are trying to get pregnant and seem to be having a problem" are useful.

– Pick a time to talk about the infertility when people are not rushed or distracted. Make sure it is a private place,

not a public place where you might feel embarrassed if you show emotion.
- Explain that infertility is considered a life crisis, and educate them about the one in five couples experiencing it.
- Tell friends and family specific things they can do to help support. It might be good to ask them to call and talk about a test or treatment, or you might want to ask them to wait until you are ready to talk about a test result.
- Explain that you may need a break from family gatherings and that it isn't about them, rather, it is about using your energy wisely.

The truth is that infertility has always been there since creation, but there is this reality we all must admit that it is on the increase by 400 per cent. And that is very, very, worrisome. For example, if a woman has a fibroid, it becomes increasingly difficult for her to conceive, and retain the pregnancy, because it goes to block the way of the child-formation, and its normal development. You now see that the possibility of conceiving with the fibroid available is remote. Then there are factors caused by societal build-ups. These includes challenges which the modern day life offers, stress, fatigue, job insecurity, and joblessness, thinking etc. Abortion too, has not helped matters. A single abortion in one's life could be faulty and thus affects her chances of either taking in or the womb retaining the pregnancy and successfully, giving birth. Then there is the problem of infections, which some people, do encounter now and then, if there is inflammatory disease, that would cause blockage and so many others alike.

Fibroid: This is a tumor, it is a growth in the womb. It grows in women. It could be in three places in the womb, like in-between the walls of the womb, that is, fleshy part of the womb. Fibroid has always been there for ages. The unfortunate thing these days is that you now see young girls, very young lames with cases of fibroid. They are all related to changes in environment, the food we eat. Today, the world's food grows on fertilizer, artificial manure, which is basically composed of chemicals. Is it cassava, chicken, vegetables, cereals, fruits, and tubers. Commercial agro output today is dependent on these formulated chemicals called fertilizers. Then environmental pollution is contributory too. And when we think of the cosmetics our women use nowadays, you quickly sum it up that there's no place to hide from such affections. Some of these bleaching agents these women use contain such heavy metals like mercury, aluminum, silicon, and compounds, like hydroquinone, are all dangerous.

Unknown to women, these elements and organic compounds enter their body - through the skin, and continue to pile up and causing various damages both inside and outside the body.

Vaginal Discharge: This can be normal or abnormal. For the purpose of this analysis, we are interested in the abnormal discharge.

Discharge is abnormal if it is excessive, offensive (smelling), yellow or green in colour, or when it causes itching. It occurs in the vaginitis, and may be caused by various micro organisms with protozoa parasite, trichonomous vaginatis cause discharges of varying colour and odour. Within the production years, of women, one of the commonest discharges is the male sperm that flow out immediately after a relationship. This is called leucorrhea, it is common within the developing countries, and it is responsible for about 30%-40% of infertility among women. The treatment depends on its cause. Infections are treated with antibiotics drug or antifungal drugs.

In the alternative therapy environment, clinically packaged, herbal medicines, are very effective, in the treatment of virginal problem. Herbal medicines have put smiles on the faces of many women previously considered, infertile.

Sexual Problem of Men:

The production of healthy sperm from the man is a condition for pregnancy. One of the major cause of infertility in women is male infertility. Azoospermia (where there is no sperm) and oligospermia (where few sperm is produced) are two of the factors that cause infertility in women because of the unhealthy nature of sperms produced by their male counter parts. Inabilities of sperm to penetrate the cervical mucous, blockage of spermatic tubes, or damaged sperm ducts are indirectly responsible for infertility in women.

Annovulation:

The failure to ovulate is a common cause of infertility in women. This can be a result of stress, hormonal imbalance or a disorder of the ovary.

Blocked fallopian tube:

Blockage of the fallopian tube due to pelvic inflammatory disease will prevent the male sperm from flowing into the eggs. In some situations, where entopic pregnancy occurs and surgery is carried out, the tube may be removed and therefore render the woman infertile.

Antibodies:

The presence of anti-bodies in the woman cervical mucous may not provide the ideal environment for the male sperm to fertilize the eggs. The sperm may be killed or become immobile. The treatment involved will be dictated by its cause. Should the male partner be responsible for the problem, the male will be treated. In situation of azoospermia, adoption of a child or artificial inssemination may be the only option. In some situation, drugs such as **Clomiphene** or **Gonadotropin in Hormone Therapy (GHT)** are applied if it is a hormonal related cause. Inability to ovulate may attract ovarian stimulation through the use of clomiphen. Blocked or damaged fallopian tubes can be taken care of through surgery or if unsuccessful, vitrofertilization approach may be adopted.

In the alternative therapy, herbal preparations, such as fruit of the womb, gamma syrup, Hercilin, U and I formula, and goncure formulae are very potent in giving total cure to infertility problem among women.

Coping with toilet disease discharge: The female genitals are naturally made to clean and defend itself. It does this by way of secreting chemical fluid that constantly "wash" and bath it out from the inside.

This fluid is naturally a bit acidic so that it can act as a defense from the would-be invading organism. The normal woman finds her pants a bit moist at the end of the day. That is as a result of her normal cleaning fluid. It should be coluorless when seen against white panties, and have a mild smell that resembles a sweaty armpit.

There should be no itching associated with this discharge, and no swelling also in the genitals. Abnormalities in the discharge of a woman should make her known that there is something wrong, and the character of the discharge and associated symptom are usually a pointer as to what organism one is dealing with.

Yeast: Also known as Candida albicans. The most common cause, of vaginal itching in the tropical regions. This is because most fungi (a class of micro-organisms) thrive in warm, humid environment, such as we have in Africa. It is also common when the patient is pregnant, diabetic, or in another state of immune compromise due to chronic disease. Candida present with white discharge that could either be lumpy or liquid, intense itching and sometimes pain from the bruising that results from itching.

There is often a yeast-like smell to the discharge and some women scratch themselves so badly, they present to the clinic with blood in the finger nails. Even though most fungi are usually stubborn, Candida is relatively easy to treat. The main stay of treatment with Candida is medication from the azole family.

Ketonazole, Fluconazole, are the generic names of drugs that treat Candida, available in oral form, as well as the form of vaginal tablets. In the case of re-current infection possible due to any of the reasons stated above, it might be necessary to put the patient on prophylactic treatment. This means giving drugs before the patient falls ill, so as to avoid the illness. Outside orthodox medicine, much has been discussed about the role of **live yoghurt** (yoghurt made fresh on the farm with all the "good" bacteria in it), and **fresh garlic** as having prophylactic, effects on vaginal yeast infection.

The things that will not cure Candida are inserting garlic into the vagina, as some texts might claim, drinking plenty of milk, stopping to drink milk, eating synthetic chalk, or the local calcium chalk rock, washing the vagina with savlon or any other kind of antiseptic.

Bacteria vaginosis: This is the second most common cause of discharge that happen in this part of the world, Africa. Bacterial vaginosis or BV for short, is one of the most distressing, to the patients, that present in the clinic, because apart from the generic symptoms, that it classifically presents with, there is a characteristic smell of spoilt fish that accompanies the discharge.

Many women come in complaining that their partners find that their personal smell is offensive and therefore want to avoid sex with them. The smell typically worsens around the time of her period, after she had just taken a pee, or just after sex.

Bacterial vaginosis presents with a colourless to creamy discharge that could be accompanied by itching in the later stages of the infection. The colour could also progress to yellow, green, and be blood, stained, although this is usually this sign of infection, with other organisms, that are considered to be opportunistic. The distressful, of the smell in BV makes patients try all sorts of remedies, The effective treatment for BV is **metronidazole** and if that name is familiar to most people, that is because, it is also the name for **flagyl**. The same remedy that could be used for diarrhoea, due to intestinal infection could be used for BV.

Trichomonas: This has a very itchy presentation, and produces a lot of discharge, so such so, that, the patient complains that her under wear gets soaked. It typically does not get so smelly like the ones listed above. Except when other organisms, colonize the place as well.

Gardenalia: Another usually seen cause of vaginal discharge that could be quite uncomfortable until identified in the laboratory and treated. It is still not as common as the earlier two exhaustively discussed.

These are the common causes of discharges due to infection in clinical presentation, but are by no means the exhaustive list. The prevention of infection of the organisms that cause vaginal discharge could be specific, the general mode of prevention include:

a. **Avoidance of nylon panties or under wear;** this is because heat and moisture from the vagina is trapped in the fabric and creates a breeding ground for the bacteria to rapidly multiply and infect the vagina.

   Practice good personal hygiene, its amazing the number of women who report wearing the same under wear for 2 to 3 days, at a go.

b. **Avoid use or over-use of vaginal douching products;** as they tend to push organism from the outside, further into the vagina.

Wash underwear, dry in the sun, to help kill off bacteria, or iron with a slightly warm iron, if you can't get sunshine.

Food Poisoning.

Food poisoning is the most misunderstood term in medical practice. In the past, anytime a doctor mentioned that a patient could have food poisoning. Negative chain reactions get in. A patient said,

- "Doctor, let me think where I ate last."
- "Doctor, this is not possible, it was my wife's food that I ate last; and she wouldn't do such a thing."
- "Doctor, I attended a dinner party, last night. You mean somebody would have deliberately, poisoned me?"
- "Doctor, I have been very careless, in the last 24 hours." I have been eating nonsense right, left and centre."
- "They have got me at last, oh my God".

Now, people are becoming more discerning, although there still exists a few ignorant few. You know, Nigeria is a dinner prone and celebration conscious society - not only do people get food poisoning by eating, contaminated food, but also the type of food and method of preparation contribute. Always avoid salad, if cream had been added, during preparation. Considering the major cause of food poisoning in Nigeria, foods are prepared early and eaten late. You know Nigeria due to lack of constant electricity is not a refrigerating nation. And we do not help matters by our lack, of elementary hygiene. Someone, who has a dinner party for say 7pm, wakes up by 5am, and starts preparing the food. Clear 14 hours before the dinner time. By 10 to 11am, all food including salad has been prepared and covered.

And the ignorant few would add cream to the salad, forgetting that the cream automatically becomes, a culture medium, for micro-organism, which will incubate then for 8 to 10 hours before the dinner is eaten. Stated below are some standard guidelines for people going for late dinner.

a. Avoid salad if cream has been added to it. Eat salad only when you add cream yourself.
b. As much as possible, avoid wet foods, if the method of preservation is suspect.
c. If the dinner is too late, do not eat heavily.
d. If the dinner is too late, please, take a lot of fluid in form of water, with your meals, in case there would be food poisoning.
e. Avoid, temporarily re-warmed food the re-heating must be constant.
f. As much as possible, limit the number of food combinations you take. You gain nothing by tasting the various types of food on the dinner table.
g. Do not be greedy, if you eat much you purge more.

Also for dinner hosts, follow this guidelines;

a. Do not start early to prepare your food, if the dinner is going to be late.
b. Do not put cream or pastes into your salad or sandwich, let the people put the sauces on the consumption.
c. Avoid activities that would delay the dinner, eat the dinner early, and activities later,
d. Get professional help, so that you could re-heat your food constantly, and not temporarily.
e. Do not put more than one type of food in a serving bowl.
f. Let scrupulous hygiene be maintained when preparing the food, and around the food.
g. Observe your workers or any persons that visits the toilet more than twice in an hour, should be excluded from the food preparations.
h. The food should not be displayed near the lavatory.
   All these guidelines mentioned above will help reduce food poisoning to the barest minimum in our society.

What is food poisoning?

Food poisoning is ingestion of bacteria by eating contaminated food. It is a common cause of diarrhea and vomiting.

A history of a recent suspect meal supports the diagnosis. The food eaten, incubation period and clinical picture give clues as to the causative organism. Certain organisms are known to be pre-dominant in certain types of food and this guides the doctor during history taking to pin-point the type of organisms and the drugs to administer, example;

- If vomiting and headache are the dominant feature, the symptoms, usually occur ½ to 6 hours, the type of food could be beef, salad, or poultry. The organism is staphaureus enterotoxin, and is heat stable.
- If vomiting only is dominant and occurs 1 to 6 hours, rice is usually the food and organisms are bacillus cereus, enterotoxin, survives boiling,
- For diarrhorea, vomiting and abdominal pain, which occurs at 2 to 48 hours, then salmonella organism which is heat stable is implicated.
- For a bloody stool associated with abdominal pain which comes 48 to 120 hours, then poultry is implicated and Campylobacter jejuni is the organism.

Management:

- Most cases of food poisoning are self-limiting.
- Give oral fluid - oral rehydration therapy.
- Antibiotics are seldom indicated but should be considered, if campylobacter causes prolonged, severe abdominal pain or relapses, (Erythromycin 500 mg 6 hourly may be considered) Ciprofloxacin is also good. The best prevention is for all dinners to be eaten wisely and correctly.

Beware food poisoning is real.

Sometimes, one finishes a meal, and finds himself in a hospital. There are even some, who are not so lucky. And before help can ever reach such people, they are dead. What causes the death? Food poisoning.

If you really want to prevent food poisoning in your home, you have to be very careful with foods, like meat, poultry, seafood, and other related food items. This is because, sometimes, the bacteria, cling to these food items. Therefore, right from when you are buying your meat or storing them in your freezer, you should be careful to separate them from other food items. Especially those ones, you are likely to eat without cooking for long or cooking them at all. The meat and poultry should be properly cooked. Also never forget to wash your hands, cutting boards, dishes, and utensils, with soap and hot water both before and after they are in contact with raw meat, poultry, or sea food.

If possible, use separate cutting boards, for animal products and other non-animal or sea foods. Always place cooked food on a dish that you know is absolutely clean. A great number of food poisoning, stem from apparently clean looking dishes, that were actually contaminated by raw animal food, that had been placed in them before. Either freeze your food or keep it warm in the oven. Keep foods either hot or cold. The bacteria that cause spoilage and food poisoning grow best, when food is Luke-warm. As a matter of fact, food left out at room temperature for more than an hour should not be eaten.

When you want to refrigerate a hot dish, first leave it in a cool spot with the lid ajar so that it can cool down, before you put it in the refrigerator. If you put a hot dish in the refridgerator, before it cools, it will warm up the refrigerator, and endanger, everything else in it.

What more, don't ever ignore those colours of blue, and green, in your food. Layers of these colours usually indicate the formation of deadly fungus. Dairy products like milk, and yoghurt are most likely and easily vulnerable to harmful fungi. Even your breads, vegetables, and fruits are vulnerable it is always safer to eat your food fresh as they come. You should also avoid puffed, bloated or leaky can of food. Food cans are puffed up, when harmful microbes, working inside produce enough poisonous gases to swell the container. Deadly food poisoning attacks, like botulism may result, if you consume from such cans. Then, you should also be careful with your vegetables, as some raw vegetables, carry larvae of dangerous worms. While it might be tempting to munch on raw celery, or fresh carrots, experts will insist on first washing them in a solution and some safe-to-eat disinfectant. You can even use vinegar as a disinfectant.

Pesticides such as bug killers, roach poison and rodent bait are dangerous. If you use them make sure there is no uncovered food they can get into. Be sure they are not accessible to children or pets. Store carefully, and preferably not in the kitchen.

Beware of food poisoning at occasion events and parties.

When there are general parties like Christmas, there are excessive eating, people simply eat and eat till their systems can take no more. And sometimes after the celebrations not a few people end up in hospitals complaining of one illness or the other. Most times, the problem is food poisoning. And what exactly is food poisoning? It is an acute food-borne gastrointestinal infection caused by food contaminated by harmful bacteria that results in symptoms, such as diarrhea, abdominal discomfort, or cramps, and fever. And that the risk of it occurring increases with the hot weather, like we experience presently. And how does one know that he or she has food poisoning? Food poisoning most commonly manifest with frequent stooling, other symptoms include nausea, vomiting, and stomach pain.

These illness are often accompanied by fever, muscle aches, shivering, and the feeling of exhaustion. These micro-organisms that cause food poisoning, can enter the body in two ways:

a. First, through the food. If the food is not thoroughly cooked, the microorganisms could still be alive. This is often the case with barbecued food, for example. That means one has to be very careful with the suyas, asun, (barbecued goat meat) and the likes.

b. Second, on the food, this occurs, for example, if the persons preparing, the food do not wash their hands before handling the food.

So how should you treat food poisoning?

Most infections last 24 to 28 hours, during which, fluid is often lost from both ends. Therefore, to prevent dehydration, drink plenty of boiled water, and use re-hydration powders, if the symptoms continue.

Always in your best interest quickly get to hospital and avoid self-medication. This is because untreated or not properly treated food poisoning can lead to death.

Most time, anti-biotic treatment is necessary, but, this can only be determined by testing for microorganism responsible. And because of how deadly food poisoning can be, people should really be careful how and where they eat, especially during the festival period, when many are likely to eat out. It can be suggested that people should be extra careful, when eating meals prepared by other people at a period like this. This is because you can't see evidence of food poisoning in any meal unless of course, the food is down right stale or even rotten.

It is especially important, that anyone whose work involves handling or preparing food stays away from work, while they have symptoms to avoid passing the illness to others.

However, many people can inadvertently put themselves in trouble, not because, they are not hygienic, but because the way the food is prepared and eaten. Many of us usually eat without vegetable, and this is not good. Even if you are eating any of the Nigerian food, like yam, rice, eba, amala, pounded yam or plantain, just ensure that you put a lot of vegetables in it, and you won't have problems.

The vegetables like ugu leaves, which are very good, can be prepared, with a little vegetable oil, onions, and any brand of seasoning. And they can also make their own salad, that way, they will be sure of the source.

Furthermore, people should minimize the amount of oil they put in their food. You know there is too much oil in the system, it can make one constipate, and this can be mistaken for food poisoning when in reality it is not.

The issue of salad is very important. So people should be very careful when eating it especially when it is prepared by other people if possible, they should avoid eating salad outside their home. Or at least, they should avoid eating, it when the cream has been mixed with it, previously. You know it has eggs, and with the cream and it, it will simply heat up and cause problems, in the system. Other meals to be wary of eating, if they did not make it themselves, include fish, beans, and its products.

People should always drink enough water, sweet drinks should not be taken, in excess. People should reduce the amount of sweet drinks and each time they take those sweet drinks, they should take an equivalent amount of water to dilute it in the system. The children should not be over indulge simply because it is a party. Whatever we do, we should remember that all these things store up in the system, so the children should not just eat, without control because, it is a festive period. And anything they are given should be complemented with vegetables, and fruits.

On preventing food poisoning, the tips below will help:

a. Always wash your hands thoroughly before preparing food, after going to the toilet, and after handling pets.
b. Keep kitchen work surfaces clean.
c. Make sure food is defrosted completely before cooking.
d. Keep pets away from food.
e. Ensure food is cooked thoroughly before eating. Meat shouldn't have any pink bits.
f. Serve reheated food hot. That means, you should not allow food you have reheated to cool before serving.
g. Keep raw meat and fish covered and store at the bottom of the fridge.
h. Keep raw food covered.
i. Rinse fruit and vegetables under running water before eating.
j. Throw away any food that's past it's use by date, doesn't smell right and/or has fungus on it.

Medicinal Tips

a. **Lemon grass:** Botanically known as Cymbopogon is a genus of about 55 species of grasses. It is a tall Perennial grass. Common name include, lemon grass, barbed wire grass, silky heads, citronella grass, fever grass, or Hierba Luisa amongst many others. Lemon grass is native to India. It is widely used as herb in Asian Cuisine, and also for medicinal purposes in Africa. It has a citrus flavour and can be dried and powdered, or used fresh. Lemon grass is commonly used in teas, soups, and curries, it is also suitable for poultry, fish and seafood. It is often used as a tea in African and Latin American countries. e.g. Togo, Mexico, Dr Congo.

Lemon grass oil has antifungal properties citronella grass, (Cymbopogon nardus and Cymbopogon winterianus) is similar to the species above, but grows to 2metre and has red base stems. These species are used for the production of citronella oil, which is used in soaps, as an insect repellant in insect sprays, and candles, and also in aromatherapy which is famous, in Britain and Indonesia.

The principal chemical constituents of citronella, geranial and citronellol, are antiseptics, hence their use in household disinfectants, and soaps. Besides oil production, citronella grass is also used for culinary purposes, in tea, and as a flavouring.

Lemon grass oil, used as a pesticide, and preservative, is put on the ancient palm leaf manuscripts found in India, as a preservative.

The lemon grass oil also injects natural fluidity into the brittle palm leaves and the hydrophobic nature, of the oil keeps the manuscripts dry so that the text is not lost to decay due to humidity.

East-Indian lemon grass (Cymbopogon flexuosus), also called cochin grass or malabar grass (Maleyalam) (Inchippull), is native to Cambodia, India, Sri-Lanka, Burma, and Thailand, while the west-Indian lemon grass (Cympopogon citratus) also known as Serai in Malay, is assumed, to have its origin in Malaysia, Indonesia people used to called it Serai too or Sereh.

While both can be used interchangeably, C. Citratus is more suited for cooking. In India C. Citratus is used both as a medical herb and in perfumes. Cymbopogon Citratus is consumed as a tea for anxiety in Brazilian folk medicine, but a study in humans found no effect.

The tea caused a recurrence of contact dermatitis in one case - lemon grass is also known as "Gavatichaha" in the Marathi language, (Gavat-grass; chaha-tea), and is used as an additional to tea, and in preparations like "Kadha" which is a traditional herbal "soup" against cough, cold etc. It has medicinal properties and is used extensively in Ancient Indian Ayurvedic Medicines. It is supposed to help with relieving cough and nasal congestion.

Anti-cancer properties: Lemon grass (Cymbopogon citratus) caused apoptosis (programmed cell death) in cancer cells. Through invitro studies, the effect of citral, a molecule found in lemon grass, is examined on both normal and cancerous cells. Using concentrations of citral equivalent to the quantity in a cup of tea (one gram of lemon grass in hot water), citral induces programmed cell death in the cancerous cells were observed, while the normal cells were left unharmed.

b. **Ewuro**, or **Bitter Leaf:** World Health Organization (WHO) scientific group, on the epidemiology, of infertility states that, inability to conceive or impregnate by a couple for a period of two years is synonymous to childlessness, and the major cause of infertility is Sexual Transmitted Diseases, (STDs), gonorrhea, syphilis, staphylococcus, and genital infection. STDs have constituted a major medical problem, especially in woman such as hostile cervical mucus, fallopian tube obstruction, pelvic inflammatory disease, and pregnancy wastage, and in men are; poor sperm mobility, testicular failure, and low or no sperm count. National academy in America, urge you to eat cruciferous vegetable, because it contain compound that have profound protective effect on the body. One of such vegetable species known is called "Ewuro" in Yoruba, bitter leaves in English, or Ewebe, meaning nutritional and medicinal vegetable. Once pot of burnt bitter leave or Ewuro, is mixed with Russian penicilline vegetable, it becomes a medicine that cures infertility related diseases.

c. **Palm oil:** Palm oil or rather red oil has been found, to offer relief in eye problems and childhood diseases, until now palm oil has been mainly associated with vitamin A. Vitamin A deficiency leads to eye malfunction, and increase infant mortality. Vitamin A deficiency is especially prevalent in Africa. Diet diversification by using locally available products, is one way to alleviate the problem. More than 250 million children under 5 years of age world wide are at risk of vitamin A deficiency that can lead to blindness. The health benefits of palm oil cannot be over emphasized. Palm oil contains active ingredients that could alleviate cough, neutralize poison and soothe skin irritation. Vitamin A has been known to prevent night blindness, and other eye problems, as well as some skin disorders, such as acne.

It enhances immunity, may heal gastro intestinal ulcers, protects, against pollution and cancer formation, and is needed for the maintenance and repair of epithelial tissue, of which the skin and mucous membranes are composed. It is important in the formation of bones, teeth, aids in fat storage and protects, against cold, influenza, and infections of the kidneys, bladder, lungs, and mucous membranes. Vitamin A acts as antioxidant, helping to protect the cells against cancer and other diseases and is necessary for new cell growth. It also slows the ageing process. Protein cannot be utilized by the body without vitamin A.

A deficiency of Vitamin A may be apparent, if dry hair or skin, dryness of the conjuctiva and cornea poor growth and/or night blindness is present. Other possible result of vitamin A deficiency include abscesses in the ears, insomnia, fatigue, reproductive difficulties, sinusitis, pneumonia, and frequent cold and other respiratory infections, skin disorders, including acne, and weight loss. The carotenoids are a class of compounds related to vitamin A acting as anti oxidants or other important function. The best known of the carotenoids is beta-carotene. But there are others including alpha, and gamma, carotene, lutein, and lycopens. When foods or supplements containing beta-carotene are consumed, the beta-carotene is converted into vitamin A, in the liver. Beta-carotene appears to aid in cancer prevention, by scavenging, or neutralizing, free radicals. Taking large amounts of vitamin A over long periods, can be toxic to the body, mainly the liver. Toxic levels of vitamin A are associated with abnominal pain, amenorrhea, enlargement of liver and/or spleen, gastro intestinal disturbances, hair loss, itching, joint pain, nausea and vomiting, water on the brain, and small cracks and scales on the lips and at the corners of the mouth.

No overdose can occur with beta-carotene, although if you take too much, your skin may turn slightly yellow-orange in colour. Beta-carotene does not have the same effect as vitamin A in the body and is not harmful in larger amounts unless you cannot convert beta-carotene into vitamin A. People with hypothyroidism often have this problem. It is important to take only natural beta-carotene or a natural carotenoid complex.

Other sources of vitamin A are animal liver, fish liver oils, and green and yellow fruits, and vegetables. Food that contain significant amounts include apricots, asparagus, beef, greens, broccoli, cantaloupe, carrots, collards, dandelion, greens, dulse, fish liver and fish liver oil, garlic, kale, mustard green, papayas, peaches, pumpkin, red peppers, spirulina, spinach, sweet potatoes, swiss chard, turnip greens, water cress, and yellow squash. It is also present in the following herbs, alfa, alfa, borage leaves, burdoce, root, cayema (capsium) chick weed, eye bright, fennel seed, hops, horsetail, kelp, lemone grass, mullein mettle, oat, straw, paprika, parsely, peppermint, plantain, raspberry, leaf, red clover, rose hips, sage, uva ursi, violet, leaves, water cress, and yellow dock. Antibiotics, laxatives and some cholesterol - lowering drugs, interfere with vitamin A absorption palm oil is about the only source of vitamin A that does not have contradiction. Eating the fresh palm fruit is recommended. If you have liver disease, do not take a daily dose of over 10,000 international units, of vitamin A in pill form, or any amount of cod liver oil. If you are pregnant, do not take more than 18,000, international units of vitamin A on a daily basis, for over a month. If you have beta-carotene, because your body probably cannot convert beta-carotene into vitamin A.

d. **Honey:** Honey is one of the most valuable food supplements, its usefulness, therefore, cannot be overemphasised. In other to remain healthy all day long, we need to feed more on honey, than any other food. Remember, that John the Baptist fed on wild bee honey in the wilderness, for long and did not witness any ill health. Medical science has not neglect the importance of honey, either, take for example, royal jelly capsules that is very expensive, but contains a high quantity and quality of natural honey. It has been proved, confirmed and certified that pure honey is soothing, with antiseptic and healing properties, energy promoting, as well as good and suitable for burns and wounds. You cannot have it better than honey. In fact, honey is one of the wonders of nature and it cannot be overlooked.

Properties of pure natural honey

Pure natural honey contains, about 35 per cent protein, half of all amino-acids, and large amount of carbohydrates (natural sugar). **Essential minerals:** essential vitamins such as vitamins C, D, E, and B-complex.

Benefits of Honey

The protein content of pure natural honey is very essential for growth, and energy. It helps in the production of hormones, antibodies, enzymes, and tissues, that are essential for a healthy body. A daily intake of honey can make up for dietary deficiencies, pure honey contains half of all amino acids, essential for a healthy body. Amino acids are chemical units that make up proteins.

Pure honey gives instant energy as glucose does. If you take one or two spoons whenever tired, it will restore your energy immediately. The mineral content of pure Honey is necessary for proper composition, of body fluids, formation of blood, bones and maintenance of healthy nerves.

Pure honey contains a lot of vitamins such as vitamin-B complex C, D, and E. The micro-nutrients of these vitamins are essential to life. They contribute to sound health by regulating its metabolism. It also helps the biochemical process that releases energy from digested foods.

Uses of honey.

The delight of nature is in honey. You can use it for treatment of various ailments like asthma, ear pains, rheumatism, tuberculosis, glands atrophy of the muscles, and heart diseases.

In addition, it is use in the treatment of male/female infertility problem. Pregnancy management, cough and cold, tiredness, and weakness, indigestion, irregular, bowel movement, constipation, boils, whitlows. It is important for the management of tension and stress, miscarriages, joint pains, memory loss, and a host of other ailments yet to be mentioned.

Identification of pure honey.

Rub honey substance on a matchstick, and strike or ignite it, if it burns, then it is assumed that what you have is pure honey.

The aroma of pure honey is sweet, and different from the adulterated one. Pure honey never congeals or goes bad, and in fact, the longer it stays, the better. It doesn't leave any oily residue in a receptacle after use. If pure honey is dropped on the base of a cup, it settles down.

Pure honey mixes very well when stirred.

Marketing

On average, 85-90% of the honey consumed in the European union is destined for table consumption, where the liquid form is preferred in most countries. The remainder (10-15%) is used for industrial purposes, such as for confectionery, bakery, and pharmaceuticals,. However, Italy is the exception, with over 40% of imported honey, being used for industrial purposes, mostly, for the production of an Italian specialty called Tor Trone, which is similar to nougat. In most countries, honey of lower quality is accepted for industrial purposes only. Based on thorough research on the benefits and uses of honey, Honey is a great gift from God, to mankind, it has great export potentials, you should have a new idea, and mind set, to export this great gift of God, that is high in demand in the international market, and always have it on your dinning table. But can anybody just export honey? The answer is no, without the proper training, on how to source, package, and export. Experts are there for you, on how to go about your export business, when you decide to join, the honey making venture.

Fruits that enhance your skin

Have you used all sorts of beauty products, and yet your skin is yet to have that particular glow you have always wanted? Why not take a second look at your diet. A regime of healthy diet, with plenty water, roughages, and fresh vegetables are what you need, for a healthy and glowing complexion. Regular intake of fruits and vegetables will enhance your skin.

Below are some specific fruits and vegetables that are beneficial to the skin:

a. **Nuts:** They are good suppliers of zinc to the body.
b. **Carrots:** This will give your body the vitamin A which it needs to always keep the skin aglow.
c. **Watermelon:** This will supply your body with thiamin and vitamin B6.
d. **Oranges:** They are a good source of vitamin C. Other rich sources of vitamin C include grape fruit, pawpaw, cabbage, apple and guava.
e. **Avocados:** These are rich in vitamin E.
f. **Spinach:** These green leafy vegetables, is a good source of iron any day.
g. **Tomatoes:** These succulent red fruits are rich source of potassium. You can also get potassium in other fruits, and vegetables, like water melon, mangoes, and bananas.

It is advisable that you cut down the fat in your diet, and eat more of green vegetables especially if you have an oily skin. Furthermore, there should be low intake of fizzy drinks, tea, coffee, and especially, alcohol.

What You Should Know About Cancer.

An oncologist is an expert doctor in cancer. In the olden days, there is little a doctor can do for a woman with metastatic breast cancer, with metastatic lung cancer, and metastatic cervical cancer. Medical inactivity is then advised, looking after the woman, very well, treat her symptoms and allow her to die peacefully.

The cancer that annoys me most, or that I hate most, is the breast cancer. Why should a woman suffer or die from the mammary gland, which God gave her to feed her children? Forget the mischievous males who suck, and fiddle them for erotic pleasure. Breast is primarily a lactation instrument. A woman apart from breast-feeding does not need the breasts. Why should she then be subjected to such agony because of reproductive necessity?

Any breast lump that would develop into a cancer, if discovered early, could be removed and the woman saved. So when last did you examine your breast? Or are you embarrassed, shy, taken aback, offended or unconcerned?

What is Cancer?

Cancer is one of several disorders which can result when the process of cell division in a person's body get out of control. Such disorders produce tissue growths called "tumors".

A cancer attacks one in every four people. Cancer is a worldwide problem. It kills 4.3 million people annually. 2.9 million of them in Africa. The six most common tumors are

a. **Cancer of the liver (Hepatoma).**
b. **Cancer of the lungs.**
c. **Cancer of the breast.**
d. **Cancer of the prostrate.**
e. **Cancer of the large gut.**
f. **Cancer of the stomach.**

Although, 40% of malignant tumors can now be cured, if they are diagnosed sufficiently early, and treated appropriately. Most of the patients who consult the doctors with such advanced disease should know that the help they can give will be limited.

Although, a few tumors can be managed optimally with very limited facilities, many of the methods should be the least cost effective. However, there is something a doctor can always do even for the most hopeless patient, that is counseling, and guidance. Health screening can save life, if they work right. What a doctor does can make all the difference, when it comes to protecting our health, few advances pack the oomph of a good screening test.

Take a look at the taming of cervical cancer; is fifty years ago, the disease claimed the lives of more women each year than any other cancer. The doctors started using the pap-test, which can catch, cervical cancer, before it starts. And now, cervical cancer had dropped to number 15 on the list of killers of African women. Yet even a great screening test can have crucial weakness.

The pap-test is not perfect. Some doctors do the examination so quickly, that their patient don't get the procedure full life saving benefit. Fortunately, you don't have to lose out if you know what to do and say. Make sure you get the best from five common screenings.

How can

a. **Ovarian cancer.**
b. **Breast cancer.**
c. **Lung cancer.**
d. **Colon cancer.**
e. **Cervical cancer.**

Be diagnose? These are the five major killers, cancer wise. The good news is that if diagnosed, early, the patients, when given adequate treatment could still live his or her normal life. Why should we die early? If little screening could prolong our lives, especially for a draconian disease, the ubiquitous cancer, whose cause for now is unknown. God help us.

New Method to Detect Breast Cancer Show Promise

New test measure, water, oxygen and other breast tissues properties could be more effective than mammograms in diagnosing breast cancer.

Several types of electromagnetic waves can be used, to gauge how normal breast tissue absorbed or scattered light.

By first measuring healthy breasts, the new technique can eventually help to better understand and detect changes that could signal cancer. It is very important to know what is before you, can begin to characterize what abnormal is. The three types of waves tested included infrared light, microwaves, and low-level electrical currents. Mammograms, the standard test for breast abnormalities, use x-ray to take pictures of breast tissue. Mammograms do not work as well on dense breast and can make it easy for doctors to miss early-stage cancer in some women. Mammograms can also fail to distinguish cancerous tumours and other thick matter, raising the risk of false positives.

The new techniques measured normal tissue level of oxygen and hemoglobin, which carries oxygen in the blood. Breast cancer tissue is "more active" and uses more oxygen and blood to survive. Cells, membrane structure and the tissue's ability to conduct and store electrical charges can also be measured.

Red Wine Cuts Risk of Ovarian Cancer.

Women, who drink two or more glasses of wine a day, may reduce their risk of developing ovarian cancer. While consumption of any alcohol will slightly lower the risk of ovarian cancer, wine had the most pronounced effect, and red was better than white. After taking into considerations various factors like age, level of education, body mass, index, number of children, use of the pill, smoking and coffee intake. Alcohol provided a protective effects. This effect was caused by wine drinking, and that, women who drink beer, or spirits, got no benefits. Women who drank two glasses, of red wine daily reduced their risk of developing ovarian cancer by 85 per cent.

Drinking two glasses of white wine daily reduces the risk of ovarian cancer by about 40 per cent. This is considering taking fairly moderate alcohol, in consumption. Two drinks a day is not a huge amount.

Drinking wine increases the level of the female hormone, estrogen, especially among post, menopausal women on hormone replacement therapy.

Have you perform personal breast screening lately?

Personal breast screening exercise is paramount for every woman and it must be done on a regular basis. The essence is for you to look out for certain changes that might signal severe dangers either in the physical appearance of the breast or the way you feel, dimpling of the skin and change in the nipple.

There is need for every woman to regularly engage herself in personal breast screening.

This few minutes checklist, could be that life saving miracle.

Breast Cancer

The breast is part of the female reproductive organ that serves as one of the major attractive features of a woman. It produces milk and other immune building substances on which a new baby can be fed. Breast feeding enhances close psychological binding between mother and child. The breast is made up of glandular tissue which is separated into lobules by connective and fat tissues. It undergoes changes that are associated with the reproductive life under the influences of the female hormones. Changes takes place in the breast along with the menstrual cycle, examples are fullness, discomfort and pain and they disappear with the onset of the menstrual flow. The main female hormones are estrogens and progesterone. Estrogen prepares the reproductive organ for production and fertilization of the eggs in child bearing, while progesterone sustains pregnancy.

What is cancer? Cancer is a class of disease in which a group of cells display uncontrolled growth invasion that intrudes upon and destroy adjacent tissues and sometimes spread to other locations in the body via lymph or blood. These three malignant properties of cancers differentiate them from benign tumors, which do not invade or spread.

Cancer of the breast: Breast cancer is the most common of cancers in women all over the world. It is most common in adult women especially aged fifty years and above. It may also occur in the younger age group.

Nine out of every ten lumps found in the breast are harmless (benign). Only one in ten of breast lumps is malignant, and referred to as Breast Cancer. The commonest cause of breast lumps in the younger age group is fibroid adenoma sometimes called breast mouse. There are risk factors that initiate or facilitate the cancerous process. This could be intrinsic or extrinsic. The presence of any of all of these factors does not mean the breast cancer will develop; such a person may have a higher risk of developing breast cancer than the general population.

Intrinsic factors include:

a. **Sex:** 99% of breast cancer are seen in woman
b. **Age:** Found in middle to older age (50 years)
c. **Family history:** a woman with a positive history of breast cancer in a first degree female relation is at higher risk of breast cancer.
d. **Genetic Factor:** Certain abnormal genes (BrCa I and II) have been found in some woman who have a higher than usual occurrence of family history of breast cancer. The presence of these genes is used as a predictive factor.

Extrinsic Factor:

1. **Weight/Obesity:** Excessive weight especially after menopause is associated with a higher risk of developing breast cancer.
2. **Hormonal:** Prolonged exposure to female hormones.
3. **Others are:** Low resistance/immunity status, unhealthy diet/ nutrition and lifestyle, exposure to ultraviolet radiation.

Signs and Symptoms

The commonest sign of breast cancer is a lump in the breast or the armpit. Others include: - recent change in size of breast, a rash around the nipple. A lump/thickening in the breast that is different from the rest of breast tissue, constant pain in the breast, lump and swelling lump in the armpit or above the collarbone, breast skin looking like an orange peel, unexplained discharge from breast particularly when it is bloody.

Screening:

In order to detect breast cancer, there is need for routine breast examination. Below are the list of the breast examinations

(a) Self-breast examination.

(b) Clinical breast examination by trained health worker.

(c) Mammograph special X- ray of the breast.

(d) Ultrasound scan use of sound waves to detect lumps.

(e) Fine needle aspiration for histology.

(f) Excision biopsy and histology.

(g) Genetic testing to test for Broca I and II.

Regular screening is advised in order to pick disease early. These are some factors that can be controlled in order to prevent breast cancer, they are:-

(a) Diet and Nutrition: Fresh fruits vegetables are recommended.

(b) Maintain ideal weight to height.

(c) Avoid alcohol.

(d) Eat more of plant based foods.

(e) Stop cigarette smoking today.

Treatment of breast cancer.

1. Surgery removing the cancerous cells.
2. Chemotherapy - use of drugs.
3. Radiotherapy.
4. Hormonal/Adjunctive Therapy.
5. Complementary Therapy: side - effect includes weakness, hair/loss, etc.

Long-term or non reversible side effects.

1. Psychosexual: depression, loss of libido and anxiety.
2. Tiredness.
3. Breakdown of family relationship.
4. Loss of job.
5. Financial difficulties.

Managing side effects.

- – Maintain a positive attitude:-
- – Counseling
- – Looking good
- – Complementary therapy includes acupuncture, massage, herbal remedies, diet, and use of health supplement. These may help in dealing with depression, tiredness, and loss of appetite.

Here are the three essential steps to the great discovery.

Step one:

Stand before the mirror to do this. Place your arms at your sides, next, your arm raised above your head.

And finally, with your hands, pressed, firmly on hips and chest, muscles, contracted.

Step two:

Here, you will be lying down to look out for any change.

Put a small pillow under your right shoulder place your right hand under your head.

Use your left hand to examine your right breast.

Hold your fingers flat to feel for any lumps or thickness.

Feel the armpit. Then start on the outside edge of your breast, and feel round the whole breast in smaller and smaller circles. Finally, feel behind the nipple.

Step three:

Here, you will be looking out for bleeding or discharge from the nipple. Squeeze the nipple gently to see if there is any bleeding or discharge.

Quick Healing Strategies for Ulcer.

Every healthy person enjoys, eating, for this is one of the pleasures of life. However, people experiencing digestive disorders like ulcers, often complain of abdominal pains, among other things. Highlighted here are causes of ulcers and some healing strategies that can enhance quick healing of these abdominal wounds.

Emotional upsets and severe mental strain have been identified as common causes of gas and indigestion. However, ulcers are among the most common of all the conditions affecting the human race today. There is a peptic ulcer, duodenal ulcer as well as stomach ulcer. All these ulcers are classified as digestive disorders. But peptic ulcer occurs more frequently than many people believe or imagine. It is not peculiar to adult alone, young children may also experience it. Ulcers of the stomach however are said to be more common in women while ulcers of the duodenum or first part of the bowel are common in men. Peptic ulcer can be defined as an ulcerated or eroded area of the mucous membrane that lines all the digestive organs. It occurs most frequently in the lower end of the stomach, first, part of the duodenum, or lower end of the esophagus.

Medical practitioners say too much of hydrochloric acid (HCL) in the stomach is one of the causes of ulcer in some patients, while it has also been proven scientifically that most ulcer result from a stomach infection caused by a bacterium known as helicobacter pylori. However, ulcer are said to be rarely found in people with low levels of hydrochloric acid (HCL) in their stomach. This mean that the stronger the acid, the greater the likelihood of developing an ulcer. Other things that can cause ulcer include emotional tension, old age, anger, such as those brought on by family arguments. Arguments also seem to play an important role in the development of ulcers.

There may be only one ulcer, but occasionally several other ulcers may occur in the same patient. A patient may also have both duodenal and stomach ulcers, at the same time and when it begins, most ulcers are usually small probably less than half an inch across the duodenum and perhaps one inch across in the stomach. Ulcer especially in the duodenum, are rarely malignant, but one ulcer in every ten occurring in the stomach may be malignant.

Sign and symptoms: the common symptoms of an ulcer in all patients experiencing it is pain, which is usually sharp and severe, especially after taking some, kinds of foods like tea, coffee, alcohol. In a few cases, there can be a steady, aching or gnawing sensation, in the upper abdomen of the patients.

In duodenal ulcer, there could be complains of pains, which usually happens when the patient is hungry. The pain may even be more severe that the patient would cry. The pains may also be experienced at night, strong or painful enough to awaken the patient.

The pain can be made worse after taking some types of foods, therefore, things like alcohol condiments, seasonings, coffee, are some of the things that duodenal ulcer patients are usually advised to avoid. In some patients, the ulcer may give them an impression that it has gone and may not be noticed, or felt for several weeks, or months, but only to resurface or flare up. Again after taking alcohols, cigarette, strong wine, or even when the patient get seriously annoyed over some trivial issues or hot arguments

This means, ulcer patients should avoid emotional strain, fight or unnecessary annoyance. Another common symptoms associated with an ulcer is heart burn or inflammation of the esophagus. Too much of acid or high concentration of hydrochloric acid (HCL) can spill up into the esophagus because of the spasm in the stomach, this perhaps, can also lead to the development of an ulcer or even aggravate the situation. For ulcer to be properly treated, a contact diagnosis in hospital is needed first, that is an x-ray of both the upper and lower gastrointestinal tract would have to be done to locate where the ulcers are located within the digestive organ. The reason for proper diagnosis, and x-ray, is that, the exact location and size of the ulcer is very important for treatment purposes, especially if the ulcer is in the stomach.

For instance, if the ulcer is very large, that portion of the stomach may have to be treated comprehensively and carefully. Under certain circumstances, the portion of the stomach may have to be treated specially, particularly when the doctor suspect malignant growth or cancer in or around the ulcerated area.

Also, if there is bigger change in the size of the ulcer or say the ulcer is getting larger in spite of medical treatment, your physician may ask you to undergo surgery. But if there is an improvement in the healing process for after medical treatment, the doctor may prescribe comprehensive or further trial of treatment until the spot heals completely.

However, large duodenal ulcer should also be treated under the strict supervision of a competent medical doctor, particularly if the patient is experiencing bleeding. The goal of any ulcer treatment is to heal the internal wound and prevent it from re-occurring.

Ulcer Treatment

Treatment usually involves both mental and physical rest to allow the stomach to heal apart from the drugs like **cimetidine**, **gelusil**, **omeprazole** etc, that would be given to the patient, all the doctors agreed that ulcer patients should embark on comprehensive treatment coupled with bed rest to ensure fast healing, process. Often, if repeated, x-ray fails to show normal healing within the stomach after some periods, the trouble may be due to cancer and the ulcerated area may have to be operated through surgery.

Ulcer patients should not embark on self medication as it is the habit of many. They must carefully guard against serious complications, the worst being perforation of the ulcer, followed by severe hemorrhage and shock.

Diet is also very important in the treatment of any type of ulcers. Some doctors advises that milk should be the delight of ulcer patients. This is because it provides both protein and calcium in adequate quantities to aid healing process, and support the whole system. Taking milk may not be advisable. Milk contains calcium, and when consumed releases this calcium, which predisposes the stomach to ulcer. Therefore, your doctor will also prescribe the appropriate medications, that have soothing, healing effects on the digest systems. But patient not responding to good treatment are often advise by doctor to have surgery. One of such surgery is what is called Pyloroplasty and Vagotomy operation. Another type of ulcer surgery is called subtotal gastrectomy. Ulcer patients should not wait for treatment until a stage when they may be troubled with vomiting of blood and tarry stools, which are usually, due to the presence of hemorrhagic gastritis. Untreated ulcers for long period of time may also cause serious hemorrhage into the stomach or duodenum. Peritonitis may also occur, if the ulcer is left uncared for, and has eroded clear through, thus allowing the gastric juices to spill out into the abdomen. These are all serious complications that can only be adequately treated by competent doctors in hospital.

Patients with ulcers, should always note the condition of their stools. They are counseled to regularly observe their stool, and if the stool appears dark, or black, the condition should be reported to doctor immediately.

Important Healing Strategies

All ulcer patients including those who have had surgery should never smoke. The reason is that tobacco, is an irritant and could aggravates or trigger severe complications, in the digestive organs.

Other things ulcer patients should avoid are tea, coffee, alcohol fasting, and the use of some analgesics, unless prescribed by doctors.

They should also avoid eating fried foods, roughages, chilies, or chili pepper, spices, and seasonings. If they must drink beverages, it is advisable to use milk, though some doctors do not subscribe to this, water and fruity juices.

Above all, medical doctors advises them to always have sufficient rest, avoid hot argument, with anybody, avoid any nervous tension, cultivate an atmosphere of peace, confidence, and hope with everybody, always smile and laugh, even when provoked, be tolerant, in viewing the short comings, of others and avoid all resentment. If they can observe, all these fast healing strategies, and they learn to forgive others, then these actions will not only promote quick healing of the ulcers, it would also bring satisfaction and true peace of mind, which are major principles of treatment for any ailment or diseases

Effective Diabetes Treatment for Patients.

Diabetes rates are rising in many countries around the world, use little, or no high fructose corn syrup in foods and beverages, which support findings by researchers, that the primary causes of diabetes are obesity, advancing age, and heredity.

Meanwhile, it seems like a fairly simple equation. If you eat too much, you get fat, and if you get fat you are more likely to suffer heart disease. But the process by which the current obesity epidemic could lay waste to a whole generation of youngsters before their parents is not quite that straight forward. In fact, it's the development of diabetes - A direct consequence of poor diet, and inactive lifestyle - that is the crucial factor in this deadly chain of events. There are worries that, the public's lack of understanding of this complex disease, and how it relates to what we eat, could undermine any attempts, to change children's dietary habits before it is too late. It's an area that needs a lot of work. The idea of curative medicine is easy to sell to the public, but with this, if you do something now then the chances are, you will not get this disease later in life.

It involves a less sexy approach but at the moment, there are over one million people in the United Kingdom walking round with diabetes without even knowing it. So how exactly does a fatty diet and excess weight lead to diabetes?

Insulin is a hormone produced by the pancreas. It plays a crucial role in helping the body's cells mop up glucose from our diet and turn it into energy. Think of a corridor full of doors. You need a key to unlock each door so you can put a parcel (glucose) in each room. Well, insulin is that key.

The problem is that abdominal fat release a particular protein - called TNF-Alpha - which messes up the mechanism of the lock. In other words, the body cells become resistant to insulin. The key point here is that the damaging protein, is only released by the type of fat that gathers round the waist and not, for example on the buttocks, so diet and life style are crucial. Once the pancreas senses the insulin, it is producing is not being used effectively, it compensates by making even more of the hormone. This process can go undetected for years, but is the building block for type-2 diabetes.

With cells becoming resistant to insulin, and the pancreas over-producing, there are raised levels, of the hormone in the blood. Eventually, the pancreas becomes exhausted, and can no longer produce enough or any insulin.

The pancreas cells have been producing far more insulin than in someone without diabetes, and they eventually burn themselves out. Even at this stage, you may have no symptoms at all. Some people get tired, thirsty and lack energy, but many feel nothing. Yet irreversible damage may already be under way to the heart, eyes, and kidneys. Without the insulin "key", the glucose from our diets cannot be converted into energy, and so blood sugar levels also starts to rise.

Excess blood sugar is another key factor in the development of diabetes. This combination of factors, insulin resistance, reduced insulin production and raised blood sugar levels - eventually combines to have a devastating effect on the body's vital organs. Blood pressure can go up, circulation can be affected, and problems with vision can occur. It's believed, that much of this damage is due to inflammation in blood vessels triggered by the whole process. As the lining of blood vessels becomes damaged - a process called atherosclerosis - the risk of arteries becoming blocked increases. If they do, a heart attack could be inevitable. What worries one is that, few people may understand the connection between carrying a few extra pounds round the waist in early adulthood, and the risk of life - threatening diabetes later on.

Yet the solution is simple. The most important thing is to look at limiting weight gain and by taking regular aerobic exercise of at least 30 minutes three times a week.

Young children with insulin-dependent diabetes could be given tablets instead of injections to control their condition.

A mutation in a single gene is a common cause of diabetes in new born babies. A group of drugs called, sulphonylureas, can help these children to produce insulin. The tablets are already used to treat elderly people with diabetes.

However, they had never been prescribed to children before. A small number of babies are with neonatal diabetes each year. The condition can be devastating. Some babies suffer from muscle weakness, and neurological problem such as epilepsy. They are given regular injections of insulin.

However, these are not always effective, and their development can lag. The children usually need to take injections for the rest of their life. The cause of the condition had now been found. Di-ribonucleic acid, DNA tests can be carried out on young children with this type of diabetes. Many will have a mutation in the potassium channel gene.

This mutations cause children to produce less insulin than they should, triggering their diabetes. Children with the condition can respond to Sulphonylureas. It had been shown that over one third of patients diagnosed with diabetes before the age of 6 months will have diabetes because of a change in the potassium channel gene.

Good eating controls diabetes

Eating habits are as important for medication in controlling, type-2 diabetes. These enable people to be able to control their blood sugar level. **The do's and don'ts in controlling diabetes are:**

a. Avoiding sugary foods.
b. Limiting portion sizes.
c. Eating fewer and smaller desserts.
d. Eating less fat.
e. Planning meals,

f. Eating a lot of vegetables.

g. Limiting some carbohydrates like bread, pasta and potatoes.

The don'ts all involved

a. Eating out, and include eating at buffets, chains and fast food restaurants.

b. Selecting high fat or carbohydrate foods and choosing high fat sources of protein.

This is glycemic control among people with type-2 diabetes mellitus.

Cure for Diabetes

The herb botanical name is Vernonia Amygdalum, an edible plant native to various parts of Nigeria, that has been variously used to treat malaria, skin diseases and constipation, and to maintain normal blood sugar levels.

It is called Ewuro by the Yorubas, Ityuna by the Tivs, Onugbo by the Igbos, Atidot by the Ibibios, Oriwo, by the Edos, Chusar Doki by the Hausas in Nigeria languages, and Bitter Leaf in English.

The compounds of the present invention may bring about cell regeneration as trials involving hyperglycemic mammals have resulted in the restoration of complete insulin activity within six months.

It is thought that these compounds enhance insulin sensitization and may replace insulin, whilst initiating beta cell generation. All people with diabetes should eat right, exercise, adequately, and use drugs with well proven efficacy and safety. The scientifically proven cases of cure for diabetes are one that follows certain operations called bariatric surgery or islet cell transplant. Bariatric surgery (an operation carried out to induce weight loss in excessively fat people) is now known to lead to a cure in very fat people with diabetes, while islet cell transplantation, in which cells that produce insulin are transplanted to people with type 1 diabetes, has also been shown to cure the diabetes, at least for a few years.

Staphylococcus

Staphylococcus are any pathogenic bacteria, parasitic to human, that belong to the genus staphylococcus, the spherical bacteria cells (cocci) typically occur in irregular clusters (Gr. Staphyle - bunch of grapes), the term staphylococci is also sometime used loosely for the cluster arrangement, itself and broadly for any bacteria with such a growth pattern. The pigments produced by staphylococci are the basis of the names given to the various strain, those with colours ranging from orange to yellow are designated. Staph aureaus. They produce infection in any organ of the body such as staph pneumonia of the lungs, brain access etc. The most common food poisoning is brought by staph contaminated food. The staph organisms also generate toxins and enzymes that can destroy both the red and white blood cells. Twenty-seven species of staphylococcus are majorly identified, but the most common and most disturbing specie of these infections are staph epidermidis, which attacks the skin, and staph saprophyticus which attacks the urinary tract, and staph aureaus which destroys the immune systems, leading to numerous opportunistic infections. Staphylococcus attacks several organ of the body leading to staphylococcus pneumonia of the lungs, which leads to difficult breathing and cough condition. Staph also leads to menigitis, a condition which leads to brain abscess. Staph organisms also generate toxin and enzymes that can destroy both the red and white blood cells. Any micro organism which can go to the extent of destroying both the white and the blood cells is a serious health problem. However, for the benefit of people, staphylococcus, aureaus damages the immune system leading to joint and muscular pains, staph aureaus also attacks the blood thereby leading to crawling and pinching sensation on the skin, staph attacks the bones, the muscles, and joints leading to general body weakness. Staphylococcus also attacks the ovary, the womb and at times leading to tribal disease and blockage, and therefore leads to female infertility. Certain medical analysts believe that this infection and other categories of infection could lead to hormonal imbalances thereby leading to a change in the menstrual cycle, scanty menses, and amenorehea, where there is no menses at all. Staphylococcus could affect the sperm mortility and viscousity, thereby leading to oligosperma or azospermia, where there is no sperm at all, and therefore leads to male infertility. It demonstrates the level of the growth manner of this infection. Staphylococcus attacks, virtually, and if not every tissue and organs of the body. Staphylococcus are now resistant to certain antibiotics. Staphylococcus are bacteria infections. They are not viral infections. Research on certain herbs have helped in treating staphylococcus. Staphylococcus can be destroyed and eradicated from blood streams and other organs where affected. Couples who could not have children have taken these herbs, and conceive children, those who are disturbed by these infections have been treated. Patients on emergency situation as a result of staphylococcus have recovered and stay alive after taking these herbs. The herbs have been very reliable, remedy for treatment, of staphylococcus, skin irritations, sexual malfunctions and lost menstrual cycles have been restored, while patients are on these herbs in a short while. Itching associated with this infection can also be relieved, while the systems are totally cleared of this bacteria infection.

Hypertension Risks

Drinking four cans of caffeinated sodas a day could be raising ones risks of high blood pressure. Soda contributes to obesity. Soft drinks add more calories to the diet. The frequent hypertension among black youth is rising, and they have higher systolic blood pressure number than white adolescents. Hypertension can lead to stroke, heart failure and kidney damage.

Caffeine is considered a preventable risk factor for hypertension and cardio, vascular disease, it is estimated that 68% per cent of boys and 62%, per cent, of girls, aged 12 to 17 drink at least one soft drink a day. With a lower number, drinking coffee or tea. In a study, 81 black teens and 78 whites were put on sodium controlled diet for three days, and then made choices from a menu of food and drinks, they would consume over three days. Based on their choices, they were categorised into three levels of caffeine intake. Blacks who consumed the most caffeine, more than 100 milligrams a day - or the equivalent of four 12-ounce sodas, or four cans - had higher systolic blood pressure reading than all others in the study including whites in the highest caffeine intake category. Their average systolic blood pressure was 199.3, while a healthy young adult has a blood pressure of 160/75.

While blacks are more likely to have high blood pressure in general, the study did not show a significant differences, between blacks and whites in other caffeine intake categories.

Life Saving news about Strokes

Strokes kill more than 50,000 Nigerians each year, and disable hundreds of thousands more. It doesn't have to be that way. Immediate treatment greatly improves the chances of surviving a stroke because many drugs must be administered within 24 hours. Yet more than 50 per cent of victims did not go to a hospital within 24 hours. **One reason:**
Most people don't recognise the

a. Symptoms which may include paralysis and loss of sensation down one side of the body.
b. Dizziness.
c. Problem with speech or vision.
d. Clumsiness.
e. A sudden excruciating headache, is it possible to prevent strokes? Perhaps. To reduce your risk, exercise regularly, don't smoke, avoid, excess stress, keep cholesterol levels low.

Aromatherapy relieves pain.

Aromatherapy is use for pain relieving. Aromatherapy is effective because it works directly on the Amygdala, the brain's emotional, centre. This has important consequences, because the thinking part of the brain can't inhibit the effects of the scent. Meaning you feel them instantaneously. Of the many uses of aromatherapy, pain relief, is only one, anxiety reduction and rejuvenation are other common objectives. Aromatherapy was is an alternative methods to expedite recovery time and reduce anxiety in heart patients. It is recommended that using drops of an essential oil, such as lavender, chamomile or eucalyptus, diluted with 10z (2 table spoon) of a carrier or neutral oil, such as almond, avocado, or jojoba, dabbed, directly on the skin. This means you literally have scented relief on you. When you need it.

You don't have to limit yourself to essential oils. Limiting the length of your exposure to certain scents, however, will ensure they remain effective. Short-term exposure is the key, because people stop responding to scents after a few minutes. **To use aromatherapy for pain relaxation and rejuvenation.**

Relax: Vanilla, subjects who smelled vanilla, while completing, stress tests, had more stable heart rates and blood pressure readings than those who took the tests in an unscented environments.

Try: Place a few drops of vanilla, extract on to a handkerchief and carry it with you throughout the day.

Recharge: Peppermint, jasmine, citrus. These scents make you feel more, awake. Even though these scents are pleasant, they act as mild irritants and the effects is similar to that of smelling salts.

Try: Sprinkle a few drops of the essential oil of your choice in a candle, diffuser, or dilute two drops, in 1 spoon of avocado or almond oil, then rub it onto the back of your hand.

Relieve: Green apple, the smell of green apples, reduced, the severity and duration, of migraine, headaches, and pains, and may have a similar effect on joint pain. The scent seems to reduce muscle contractions, which are the main cause of pain in migraine.

Try: For aromatherapy pain relief, eat a green apple for a snack or bathe with green apple, bath salts.

What is Prostate Enlargement?

The prostate gland is the organ that produces semen and it stays beneath the bladder surrounding, the urethra, the tube that drains urine from the bladder, when it becomes enlarged, the prostate can put pressure on the urethra and cause difficult urination and also leads to the following symptoms:

    a. Weak urine.

b. Stopping and starting, while urinating.
c. Dribbling at the end of urination.
d. Straining while urinating.
e. Frequent need to urinate.
f. Increased frequency of urination, at night.
g. Urgent need to urinate.
h. Not being able to empty the ladder.
i. Blood in the urine.
j. Urinary tract infection
k. Back and lower abdominal pain.

Effective Ways to Avoid Mouth Odour.

There is nothing as objectionable as a smelling mouth. It is not only a minus to one's personality, it also makes one to be repulsive to others. One of the most embarassing things that can ever happen to anyone is to have a bad breath without knowing it. Bad or offensive odour coming out of a man's mouth even with him knowing can erode his confidence. The same is applicable to any lady worth her onions. A lot of factors can be held responsible for this anomaly which can be a serious source of social stigmatization. It is very easy to detect bad breath. To know if you suffer from bad breath, lick the inside of your wrist and smell the spot licked, whatever odour you perceive is your breath.

Considering the factors responsible for bad breath, food intake has a lot of effect on one's breath, a lot of people suffer from this anomaly, without knowing. The breakdown of food particles in and around your teeth can cause a foul odour. Eating foods containing volatile oils, is another source of bad breath, onions, and garlic are the best known examples, but other vegetables and spices also can cause bad breath. After these foods, are digested, and the pungent, oils are absorbed into your blood stream, they're carried to your lungs and are given off in your breath untill food is eliminated from your body. Alcohol behaves in the same fashion, though alcohol itself has almost no odour, however, the characteristic smell on your breath is mainly the odour, of other components of the beverage.

Other causes of bad breath include dry mouth, and mouth, nose, and throat, conditions, which are not limited to dental problems.

Poor dental hygiene and periodontal disease can be causes of bad breath. If you don't brush and floss daily, food particles remain in your mouth, collecting bacteria and emitting hydrogen sulphur vapours. A colourless, sticky film of bacteria (plaque) forms on your teeth. If not brushed away, plaque can irritate your gums (gingivitis) and cause tooth decay. Eventually, plaque-filled pockets can form between your teeth and gums (periodontitis), worsening this problem - your breath.

Dentures that aren't cleaned regularly or don't fit properly also can harbour odour-causing bacteria and food particles. A dry mouth can be a veritable source of mouth odour, because saliva helps, cleanse and moisten your mouth. A dry mouth enables dead cells to accumulate on your tongue, gum and checks. These cells then decompose and cause odour. Dry mouth naturally occurs during sleep. It's what causes "morning" breath". Dry mouth is even more of a problem if you sleep with your mouth open. Some medication as well as smoking can lead to a chronic dry mouth, as can a problem with your salivary glands.

Bad breath is also associated with sinus infections because nasal discharge from your sinuses into the back of your throat can cause mouth odour. A child with bad breath may have a foreign object lodged in his or her nose. A bean, or small item stuck in the nose can cause persistent nasal discharge and a foul odour. Strep throat, tonsillitis, and mononucleosis, can cause bad breath until the throat infection clears. Bronchitis and other upper respiratory infections in which you cough up odorous sputum are other sources of bad breath. Cancer sores may be related to bad breath, especially if they accompany periodontal disease. Other disease like kidney failure, and lung infections can trigger foul mouth odour.

Chronic lung infections and lung abscesses can produce very foul-smelling breath, - kidney failure can cause a urine-like odour, and liver failure may cause fishy like odour. People with uncontrolled diabetes, often have a fruity breath odour. Chronic reflux of stomach acids from your stomach (gastroesopageal reflux disease or gerd) and a slight protrusion of the stomach into the chest cavity (hiatal hernia) also can produce bad breath.

Tobacco smoking, can further, aggravate bad smelling mouth, as smoking dries out your mouth odour. Tobacco users are also more likely to have periodontal disease, an additional source of bad breath.

How to avoid bad breath:

a. Brush your teeth and tongue after you eat. Keep a tooth brush at work to brush after eating.
b. Floss at least once a day. Proper flossing removes food particles, and plague from between your teeth and tongue.
c. Brush your tongue. Giving your tongue a good brushing remove dead cells, bacteria and food debris. Use a soft-bristled tooth brush, and brush your tongue with at least five to fifteen strokes. Pay particular attention to the middle third of the tongue, where most of the bacteria tend to collect.
d. Clean your dentures well, if you wear a bridge or a partial, or complete denture, clean it thoroughly at least once a day or as directed by your dentist.
e. Drink plenty of water. To keep your mouth moist, be sure to consume plenty of water - not coffee, soft drinks, or alcohol. Chewing gums (preferably sugarless) or sucking on candy (preferably sugarless) also stimulate saliva, washing away food particles and bacteria. If you have chronic dry mouth, your dentist or doctor may additionally prescribe an artificial saliva preparation or an oral medication that stimulates the flow of saliva.
f. Use a fairly new tooth brush - change your toothbrush every three to four months, and choose a soft bristled tooth brush.
g. Schedule regular dental check ups, at least twice a year. See your dentist to have your teeth or dentures examined and cleaned. You can teach your school-age children to brush and floss their tongues to prevent bad breath. However, don't give children mouth wash, to use, because many mouth wash products contain alcohol and can pose a risk for children if swallowed.

Dental Care

Cancer of the mouth and throat preventions: Cancer is a sudden uncoordinated growth of the body cells, and this appears in the mouth unnoticed as a small lesion either as ulcer or blister. Cancer affecting any part of the body if not detected at an early stage can spread to all parts of the body through the blood stream, and may eventually result in death. Unfortunately, demographic reports in our country on relationship between cancer and death rate are not yet established. But statistics show that most cancer cases are not detected at early stage.

Cancer of the mouth (oral cancer) includes cancers on the lips, gums tongue, salivary glands, and the roof or floor of the mouth. Cancer cells growing in these areas of the mouth may spread to the lymph nodes in the neck, and into the jaw bones. Early detection and treatment are extremely important for the current forms of treatment to be most effective. Oral cancer can only be detected by a dentist, and can be detected at routine dental visit or during a dental treatment, thus millions of people are affected with cancer of the mouth, and throat, but they do not know. Prevention is not only better than cure, but also cheaper.

When oral cancer in any form is detected and treated, early, the outlook is good, resulting in a cure in three quarters of cases.

Any lump, sore, ulcer, or discolored spot in the mouth that does not go away in two-three weeks should be assessed by a dentist. Symptoms such as persistent sore throats, sore under dentures, difficulty chewing or swallowing or a lump on the neck also require medical evaluation.

What Causes Oral Cancer?

As with other forms of cancer, the direct cause of mouth cancer is not yet clear. Research continues on many fronts to find the key to way cells in various organs and tissues of the body begin a pattern of uncontrolled growth (i.e become cancerous). With mouth cancers, however, it is not known, that there are several factors that contribute significantly to their developments.

Smoking tobacco products-especially pipes and cigars (but any tobacco products can cause cancer) others are: chewing tobacco. The use of snuff, heavy alcohol, consumption, poor oral hygiene, chronic irritation of the mouth, for example, from dentures that doesn't fit well or from the broken or rough edges of teeth, exposure to sunlight (lips).

Importance of Early Detection

Your dentist has recent good news, about progress against cancer. It is now easier, than ever to detect oral cancer early, when the opportunity for a cure is great. Currently, only half of all patients diagnosed with oral cancer survive more than five years. Your dentist has the skills and tools to ensure that early signs of cancer and pre-cancerous conditions are identified. You and your dentist can fight and win the battle against oral cancer.

Know the early signs, and see your dentist regularly. You should know oral cancer often starts as a tiny, unnoticed white or red spot or sore anywhere in the mouth. It can affect any area of the oral cavity, including the lips, gum tissue, cheek lining, tongue, and the hard or soft palate.

Other signs includes a sore that bleeds easily or does not heal, a colour change of the oral tissues, a lump, thickening, rough spot, crust, or small eroded area, pain, tenderness, or numbness anywhere in the mouth, or on the lips, difficulty chewing, swallowing, speaking, or moving the jaw or tongue, a change in the way the teeth fit, together, alcohol, use combined with smoking greatly increases risk, prolonged exposure, to the sun increases the risk of lip cancer. More than 25 per cent of oral cancers occur in people who do not smoke and have no other risk factors. A diet high in fruits and vegetables may prevent the development of potentially cancerous lesions.

Regular Dental Check-up's Important

Regular dental check-ups, including an examination of the entire mouth, are essential in the early detection, of cancerous and pre-cancerous conditions. You may have a very small, but dangerous, oral spot or sore and may not be aware of it. Your dentist will carefully examine all areas of your mouth. In about 10 per cent of patients, the dentist may notice a flat, painless, white or red spot or a small sore. Although most of these are harmless, - testing can tell them apart. If you have a sore with a likely cause, your dentist may treat it, and ask you to return for re-examination. Dentists often will notice a spot or sore that looks harmless, and does not have a clear cause. To ensure that a spot or sore is not dangerous, your dentist may choose to perform a simple test, such as a brush biopsy, which usually is painless, and can detect potentially dangerous cells, when the disease is still at an early stage. If your dentist notices something that looks very suspicious, and dangerous, a scalpel biopsy, may be recommended. This usually require local anaesthesia. Your general dentist may perform this procedure, or refer you to a specialist for it.

A stitch in time saves nine-taking a proactive step against cancer of the mouth, or any other lethal disease of the body is a very wise step. It is recommended that couples take advantage of this information, and preserve their general body health. When you notice a small ulcer or blister in your mouth, that persist for more than 10 days, see your dentist very quickly for consultation and professional advice. Do not wait until the very bad stage. Be good to yourself, be proactive, and be wise. See your dentist today for the nagging ulcer.

Bacteria Worsen Asthma in Kids.

A type of bacteria could be responsible for triggering asthma attacks in children who have never experienced them before. The bacteria called mycoplasma also may exacerbate wheezing in children, who already have asthma-mycoplasma, which causes respiratory infection like bronchitis and pneumonia, seems to infect children more often than adults. About half of the children who experienced their first asthma attack were infected with mycoplasma

Many children diagnosed with asthma, suffered attacks apparently aggravated by mycoplasma infection. Mycoplasma infections are frequent, so, testing parents or siblings for mycoplasma infection could help prevent attack exacerbation in asthmatic children and may even keep children who are predisposed to asthma from having an initial attack, but, the diagnosis is rarely made because these familiar, - infections are often limited to a slight case of bronchitis or pharyngitis.

Please Stop the Polio Virus Infection in Children

Wild polio virus is a threat to the children's good health. Some got to know for the first time perhaps that polio was a viral infection, which disabled the children, occasioned by faeco-oral transmission, and prevalent among children under the age of five. It leads, eventually, to paralysis, for which no cure has yet been found. Such grim prospect, were frightening and unacceptable. A virus in medical term is a minute, terrible and infections organism that causes disease, in all life forms, but which, interestingly, depends upon a living, host for its metabolism, and replication.

Two drops of the oral polio vaccines at birth, 6, 10, or 14 weeks were all a child needed, to escape from the danger it posed. There are type 1 and type 3 cases of wild polio virus. Which is the more virulent one? Oral polio vaccine remained the best method for stopping transmission because it sterilizes even the digestive tract. Surveillance must be strongly to detect paralytic polio early, which must be reported within 14 days when detected. Besides routine immunization, supplemental immunization, which would ensure that, every child is reached. Immunization was significant because it had proved an effective preventive measure, there was abundant evidence that it brought about a reduction in child mortality, and that it was cost effective.

There are several factors that pose serious challenges to polio eradication. The first is the vaccine safety controversy which led to its rejection by a segment of the Nigeria, the second is the poor supplementary immunization activity. The third, is low political commitment of state and local councils in Nigeria. These factors informed the belief that teachers were the best agents to bring about the required change, since, pupils were more likely to believe what their teachers tell them, and since parents too, respect their opinion, in the various communities. The cultural inclinations of the north and the southern parts of the country need to be considered.

What to Know About Periods or Menstruations

If the eggs released during ovulation is not fertilized, estrogen level declines, and deprived of oxygen, the living cells of the womb begin to die. Tiny blood vessels are torn as the lining cells break away from the wall of the womb, and it is the combination of dead cells and blood from the tears that comprise menstrual flow.

In healthy women, the torn vessels, begin to clot and heal within a day or two, and bleeding slows. Usually, there are two heavy days of flows. And for most women, these occur on the second and third days of their cycle. While menstrual blood varies from woman to woman, here's a general guide.

Colour: Usually dark red, but can be bright red if it is very profuse.

Consistency: It consists of blood, degenerated cells from the uterine lining, mucus from the cervical glands and bacteria. It may contain "clouts" of mucus and endo-mentrium, which should be stringly and elastic, not bloody, when flattened.

Odour: Usually odourless, but can smell a little cheesy.

Quantity: Most people lose 20 to 80 ml (4sps to 4 tbsps) of blood over a five day cycle. If you bleed regularly for more than seven days, or soak three tampoon in two hours, contact your doctor.

All you need to know about Menopause.

Menopause is a period in the life of a woman, when there is no longer ovarian function and definitely such a woman is ageing. Menopause is that period when the normal functioning of the ovary of a woman, in terms of the production of necessary hormones that results in ovulation stops. The period of menopause varies in women. Depending on the standard of living, it could be as early as 45 to 48 years, or as late as 50 years, but generally, it is about 50 to 52 years.

Standard of living affect the early or late menopause. People who are well fed, women who takes care of themselves, those who are not involve in stressful activities have longer period, before their menopause.

Can food supplements which so many women who are yet to start menopause swallow in form of tablets help to curb the stress of menopause? There is a period a girl child start observing her menstruation. That period is called menarchy. When she starts observing her menses, it means that she had developed up to a stage and that she could get pregnant. She could now start her reproductive life. Now, the eggs are produced in the ovary and every month, one is shed in terms of ovulation. So if there is no pregnancy, there will be menstruation. And that one goes on for some time. At a particular age, in life, or a stage in life, the eggs get exhausted it is this exhaustion of the eggs from the ovary that brings about menopause. When a girl starts her menses early, her menopause starts late, while those who start late do have early menopause.

This means that some people, who starts early, are likely going to end later, and those who start late might end up faster. So, for the food supplements, they are good, vitamins minerals, are what the body needs for the day to day activities. We are suppose to get them from the food we eat, but often times, the food we eat does not supply all these. So if you can get it as supplements, why not? Food supplements do makes menopausal women feel better, but not necessarily cure menopause. Menopause is not a disease, in the first place, it is a normal psychological change, but, definitely not a disease, so food supplement cannot cure menopause.

Are there some things a lady may lose at menopause apart from her menses? At 13 or 14 years, when a girl starts observing her menstruation, is another stage, Now appearing with this stage are some changes which distinguish her as a female in shape and in voice, for instance what brings about those changes are the emergence of some prominent reproductive hormones. At menopause, when those reproductive hormones are no longer there, definitely these advantages that she has had cease to be. What are those advantages that cease to be at menopause? First of all, a lady can loose her figure. It is the reproductive hormones. That gives a woman the right shape of a woman. The development of breasts, good curves, and so on.

So, what happens when all the hormones are no longer there due to menopause, is that, all the feminine areas will shrinkle. A woman may now have flat breasts, her buttocks, could become flabby, her vagina that is normally moist because of reproductive hormones will be dry. That is why menopausal woman complain that sexual activities at that stage are injurious.

How about hot flashes that so many menopausal women complain of? Hot flashes are experiences that a woman in menopause or around menopause undergoes. It is more prominent among the whites than in blacks. White woman have reddish patches due to hot flashes. In blacks, you don't see the reddish patches, but, then there are some attitudinal changes that blacks experience. Some will become so easily agitated mood changes, will be there. Some may not be able to sleep at a particular time. And that is way sometimes, some menopausal women are placed on what is called hormone, replacement therapy. For those that cannot bear it. But, because, it is a psychological thing. It is what every woman should be able to bear, because after some time, the hot flashes, and menopausal stress get subsided.

There are some dangers of menopause. The dangers are expressed in osteoporosis which means the wearing away of bones, at this stage, a menopausal woman is not suppose to be involved in strenuous works. Then for vagina dryness, can something be done to bring back its moisture? Yes, and that is what is called hormone replacement therapy. In the absence of the reproductive hormones that makes vagina moist. If the dryness is more than what the person can bear, she can have the hormones, in form of tablets.

But, how about the side effects of these hormonal tablets? Yes, there are side effects of course. There is nothing one does that does not have side effects. But, I don't like talking about side effects, often, because there is actually nothing you do in life without side effects really. So, what is beneficial to another person, so each patient is individualized and if you think you are having some feeling that you cannot explain, may be the best person to actually decide for you is your doctor. Your doctor will be able to enlighten you on what you need to do. But, it is surprising that some women get pregnant at the first stage of menopause. A certain woman went to the hospital for pregnancy test at her early stage of menopause, and she was shocked that the result of the pregnancy test was positive. But how could that be? The truth of the matter is that since menopause has set in, the functioning of the ovary has stopped. Eggs are no longer produced then there is nothing for the sperm cells to fertilize, and therefore there is no pregnancy. Those are two extreme that I am are talking about, I am talking about that time when a woman is in the normal reproductive life, and she is producing eggs. And I am talking of another time when the eggs are no longer there, and she is not producing anything.

If that is the case, how do one explain the case of that certain woman? Yes, in between the period a woman is still observing her menses, and that of her menopause, there is a period where a woman is not actually yet in menopause, but she is already drifting away from the normal menarchy. They call it perimenopause, period. At this period, menopausal period, the shedding of eggs may not be constant, or coming every month. But pregnancy can occur. But, by the time you get into full menopauses there will be no pregnancy.

For menopausal women out there, and those on the verge of menopause, every woman should know that there is always a beginning and an end to everything. Menopause is just an end to menses and should not scare any woman.

Sex in Menopause

Menopause is the termination of the monthly menstrual flow of the female. It signals the end of a womans' reproductive cycle. While it is something to look forward to because it has the advantage of bringing the inconvenience associated with menstrual flows, to an end. It also comes with complications like mood swings, hot flashes, and sexual irritation. However, ageing is not the only cause of menopause can also result as a side effect of some surgeries. For instance, the surgical removal of ovaries due to growths, infection, tubal pregnancy or the removal of the ovaries in the case of permanent family planning method may bring about early menopause.

Menopause, has also been observed to result early from the usage of some cancer drugs. There is another type of menopause called the "cold turkey", this occurs following an abrupt stoppage of menopausal hormonal therapy. The age when menopause begins in women vary depending on some peculiar predisposing factors such as environment, health, diet, genealogical differences, and so on. Generally, though menopause, can occur between the ages of 45-55. Though the menstrual cycle will not stop abruptly in most ladies. It first becomes irregular and then lengthens. Ovulation may also become irregular. When this happens, a woman will observe that she experiences, hotness of the upper part of the body, restlessness, and intermittent sweating. The most disturbing aspect of this menopausal visitation for most women is that the female sexual organs begin to experience a down turn in appearance, the organs begin to lose their freshness and sparkle. A woman will also notice some degree of atrophy, especially in her breasts, and her vagina. Her vagina, for example, will be unusually dry sometimes. The loss of the organs freshness and vigour could also make the genitals to be prone to infections. This loss of freshness may be, due to the reduction of estrogen, in the body. Now, how does all this affect a woman's sexual life? Well, when these sudden changes are not prepared, for and accepted with equanimity, they may do a great deal of damage to her sense of worth and sexuality.

Women who don't prepare for menopause usually battle with doubts, and they end up seeing themselves as being unable to maintain an active sexual life.

They think they can no longer sustain their sexual activities and they may even give up on their sex lives. Others think that since their husband's sexual drive still seem to be the same, they may loose them to younger women.

Pregnancy After Menopause

Some years ago, a remarkable study showed that women who had gone through menopause as long as two years previously could become pregnant using donated eggs. Four of the seven women gave birth to healthy infants, one had twins, in fact.

The donated eggs came from healthy young women and were fertilized with sperm from the menopausal women's husbands.

At the same time, the menopausal women were given hormones to stimulate a menstrual cycle in sync with that of their donors. Further good news: The technique also may work for women in their fourties who though not past menopause, have not been able to conceive normally.

A New Contraceptive

Norplant, the first really new contraceptive in years, sounds almost too good, to be true. It is a series of capsules containing the hormone progesterone, implanted, just under the skin, usually in the upper arm. It's 99 per cent effective and doesn't need to be replaced for 5 years. If a woman does want to become pregnant, it can be removed at any time, and fertility will resume immediately. It's safe, require no daily effort or sexual restrictions and the only major side effect is menstrual irregularity.

Do you know that Snoring can lead to Premature Death.

Snoring can pose a lot of serious health and social hazard to anyone who fall victim. A woman almost call her marriage quit, after discovering that her husband snored in a commercial bus they boarded, with friends after attending a night party. The man started vibrating the vehicle with snoring publicly. The woman said, he does snore anytime he sleeps, and according to her, she hates men who snore, and she had always warm her hubby that unless he stop snoring, she will not marry him, but the husband thought his wife is not serious. She said maybe he thought she was joking. She said as the bus started, moving that night, her husband yawned and leaned against the back of the bench in the front row. She never thought he was going to sleep, otherwise she would have cautioned him. The bus was filled with passengers and everybody was silent. About five minutes, later, the husband broke the silence, snoring very heavily like a cow. He drew everybody's attention and some passengers burst into laughter, while some kept hissing, and watching him with disgust. The most painful thing to her was that her friends were also with them in the bus, she almost ran mad with anger. On reaching their destination she told him to keep away from her, and that she doesn't want to have anything to do with a snorer.

Snoring is noisy breathing, through the mouth or nose during sleep. Snoring is something that virtually every one does occasionally. Wife might stop sleeping in the same room with her husband. This is really causing a serious problem between them now. Snoring often constitutes a social embarrassment, and a nuisance to the sleeping partner of the person that snores. Though, the woman's husband snoring habit may not be the only reason the woman has decided to severe the relationship.

Many partners of snorers decide to sleep in separate rooms, and the resulting lack of bedtime chat, and physical intimacy can lead to a strained relationship. The snorer often becomes isolated and frustrated, about a problem they seemingly have no control over. Relationships often suffer as a result of snoring. The sleep partner of a snorer may resort to sleeping in a separate room, which changes the dynamics of bedtime. Snoring thus affects the physical and social intimacies of a relationship. The snorer feels isolated, and both partners are unhappy. Snoring has always been a part of the reasons why some couples break up. Snoring cannot be the only reason for which marriages or relationships collapse, but it definitely contributes to it.

People snore when they are congested. Even the baby or a beloved pet may snore. In this cases, it is not a problem, but snoring is a problem, if you stop breathing, during sleep and have to wake up to catch your breathing. You are disturbing your sleep because of your snoring. The psychological pains of snoring is only felt by the snorer's sleeping partners.

I don't know of any psychological factor that can make a person to snore habitually. But whoever sleeps close to a snorer, feels the impact. Such a person may not be able to contain the pains and he becomes very uncomfortably disturbed. As a results, he may raise a protest that leads to a perpetual fight.

Snoring is not just a social embarrassment, and a nuisance to a sleeping partner, it can also have a serious health consequences. Sleep and relaxation go hand in hand. During a deep sleep, the muscles in the body relax, and as the muscles in the throat relax the airway partly closes. This is normal. Air comes into and out of the lungs through this airway. However, if the air flow in the throat and nose is obstructed, the air passage is narrowed, which causes snoring. Snoring is the fluttering sound created by the vibrations of tissues, against each other can be the soft palate, the throat, the uvula, the tonsils, or the adenoids. (The soft palate is the soft part of the roof of the mouth). Snoring occurs when there is a narrowing somewhere in the air passage between the nose and the larynx. Ordinarily, it happens to anybody who lies face-up while sleeping. Especially when the person is fagged out from the day's work. In this case, the muscles of the air passage become lax and very weak, and consequently impair breathing. So, it is advisable to stop lying down while sleeping.

What about some people who lies face-down while sleeping, and yet snore very heavily? These are the people whose case calls for medical attention. Generally, fat people often fall victims, of snoring irrespective of the manner in which they sleep. The reason is that fat people suffer from what we call mucousal laxity. A man who is fat is likely to experience weakness of tissues, in his air passage, which narrows the air way and causes obstruction to breathing.

For those aware that they snore, and yet do not see it as posing a serious health attack or risk. Usually, snoring causes sleep loss for both the snorer's and their sleep partners. The snorer may wake frequently, either from the snoring or from the jostling to stop the snoring. The sleep partner has trouble sleeping deeply because of the snoring plus anxiety about their partner's health, and well being. This sleep deprivation has consequences during the day. These include sleepiness, irritability and lack of productivity.

In addition, to problems stemming from sleep deprivation, snoring can cause more serious health problems. These include daytime sleeplessness, a compromised immune system and slow healing, poor mental and emotional health. Lack of smooth functioning of the body, decreased productivity, a negative mood, low energy, unclear thinking, and slower reaction time. In addition, snoring causes reduced oxygen flow to the brain, which can lead to premature death, type II diabetes, high blood pressure, hypertension, stroke, and heart, disease. Snoring can also be a symptom of sleep apnea, that is life threatening. In explaining the meaning of apnea, if you stop breathing periodically, during sleep, you have sleep apnea. You may awake to restart breathing up to 100 times per night. Probably you remember nothing at all about the awakenings. Mild snoring hardly results to apnea. You stand the risk of having apnea, if you have severe snoring. If snoring stops when the snorer wakes up, and turn over, that is mild snoring. Severe snoring is continual snoring regardless of sleep position. If you sleep alone, you will find it more difficult to determine, if you snore a little or a lot. Some snorers, wake themselves with the noise, and know that they snore.

Other snorers are awakened by annoyed neighbours in nearby apartments banging on the wall, in the middle of the night. If you wake in the morning and do not feel rested after a reasonable number of hours, of sleeps, you may wish to see a doctor and get tested at a sleep clinic for snoring sleep partners of heavy snorers, awaken, over twenty times per hour, which severely cuts into the quantity and quantity of their sleep. The partner may try to stop the other person snoring, or they may simply, be awake, wishing they were asleep.

Snoring can be transferred through inheritance. If you inherit a narrow throat, which can cause snoring, then you snore whenever you sleep. Men are more prone to snoring than women, due to excess weight and fatty tissue in the neck, which cause their throat to become smaller. As you grow old, your throat decreases. Men have narrower air passages, than women and are more likely to snore.

Smoking relaxes muscles and also creates nasal and lung congestion. Exposure to second-hand smoke can cause the same snoring problems as smoking does. Examine your throat, nose, mouth, palate, and neck, check for underlying health conditions, possibly enroll for a test at a sleep clinic, where someone can observe, your sleep, patterns and diagnose your snoring problem, and help you to stop snoring. Unfortunately, no sleep clinic exists in Nigeria! But since finding a solution, to your snoring problem results in an improved quality of life for you and your loved ones, you can try the following, self-help tips to prevent or alleviate your snoring.

a. Loosing weight will reduce the fatty tissue in your airway. Eating less and improving your fitness level can significantly improve your ability to breathe freely, when you sleep.

b. Sleeping on your back may cause the flesh of your throat to relax into your airway, so adjusting your sleep position, can alleviate snoring. Changing your sleep position may stop mild snoring, but severe usually snore in any position.

c. Try sleeping without a pillow. Pillows can block your air way by bending your neck.

d. Placing rolled up towels under the head of the mattress is an easy way to change the angle of the mattress. Elevation of the head of your bed, may make breathing easier, and encourage your tongue and jaw to move forward. Elevating the entire head of the bed is better than using a pillow which can crimp the neck and contribute to snoring.

e. Stopping smoking can help with the noise and intensity of your snoring.

f. Limit the intake of food or alcohol before bed, do not eat or drink heavily within three hours of your bedtime. These substances relax your muscles and increase the likelihood, of snoring.

g. You may be taking sleeping pill or tranquillizer to help you sleep, but sedatives also relax your neck muscles, which can contribute to snoring.

Bleaching of the Skin

Do you know that bleaching of the skin is extremely dangerous to the health? Bleaching has become most popular amongst both males and females these days. It is also described in various ways to mask what it actually is and make it more acceptable. The term used include toning, blending of skin colour. Bleaching is usually a continous thing, once you start, you have to continue to maintain the artificial colour. This is because your natural skin colour is encoded into your genes, and your skin will always gives out that colour.

What is bleaching of the skin?

Bleaching of the skin involves the attempts to transform the colour of the skin to a lighter colour using several means. The skin consists of two layers. The outer layer-epidermis and the inner layer - dermis. A substance called melanin is responsible for the dark colour of the skin and protects us from the harmful effects of the sun. The melanin in African skin is a result of an evolutionary adaptation in our ancestors to help them survive the intensity of the sun. This is in obvious contrast to white skin found in human being in the temperate regions of the world. The method of bleaching used usually involves chemical substances whose action on the body range from harsh, abrasive to mild, and gentle. An example is hydrogen peroxide, which is used for skin peeling and alpha hydroxyl acids which also peel mildly, and are described as exfoliators. Most bleaching agents are applied topically on the skin, but more recently, tablets have been formulated to act from within.

Why do people bleach their skin?

The skin is often described as the largest organ in the body, because it covers the whole surface of the body. It is the packaging that we are wrapped in (just like when you are giving a gift). Skin bleaching may stem from a psychological feelings of inferiority as to the person's outward appearance (although it also reflects a problem from within). There is an attempt to be more acceptable by lightening the skin through bleaching. These may be to look more attractive to the opposite sex in general or a particular person (e.g. a straying husband, a new or younger lover). It may be as a result of peer pressure, especially among females. A young girl may see her friends using bleaching creams, and catch on the habit. She may see it as fashionable and trendy. A very tiny percentage of people have a skin problem, and are placed on topical steroids by a medical doctor. This is done under close medical supervision, and these steroids may lighten the skin. However, doctors usually prescribe topically steroids for only a specified period of time during which the treated condition clears. The treatment is also usually, for small and specific parts of the body affected, not the whole body!! Skin bleaching actually show insecurity about your own natural appearance. Some people believe it gives them a good, finish. It seems to be a fad that has caught on. When people decide to start bleaching, they seem not to hear the hunter's whistle. The lure of a lighter skin seems to outweigh all the possibilities of burnt or greenish skin. The origin of modern skin bleaching in itself speaks for the practice. Black women in America who wanted to be acceptable by being as white as possible, started the modern bleaching culture.

There are various types of bleaching agents, and their actions, and harmful effects on the users. Some female users, when there is need to pass through caesarian section for a child delivery, mostly finds it difficult to heal in time, or the wound can be easily infected, thus leading to a serious medical case.

Stopping Hair Loss

Men who suffer from male pattern hair loss have several options. They can either choose to chemically treat hair loss, get artificial wigs or weaves, if drug treatment is ineffective, or impossible, or invest in a permanent solution, hair transplant surgery.

Drugs: The only Food And Drug Administration, FDA approved drugs available to medically treated hair loss are, propecia (finasteride) and rogaine (minoxidil). Both products slow further thinning of hair and increase coverage of the scalp. *Propecia* inhibits the conversion of testosterone into dihydrotestoterone (DHT), a hormone that shrinks hair follicles, whereas, Rogaine stimulates hair follicle.

Neither medication, will produce full regrowth of hair and the length or texture may be slightly alter the areas of regrowth. Also, the effectiveness of medications, deperias, on the cause of hair loss, and the extent of the loss and individual response rates. Both products work best, if hair loss is recent, (within five years) and occurs on the top of the head rather than near the forehead.

Usually the drugs take at least a couple of months to produce a noticeable effects. However, these medications need to be taken continuously. If the medications are stopped, any hair that has grown in will gradually be lost, and within six to twelve months, the scalp will look the way it did prior to treatment.

a. **Wigs and weaves:** If a man has medical conditions, or allergies, that may interfere with the use of pharmaceutical solutions for hair loss or chooses not to undergo hair replacement surgery, he may opt for wig, toupes, or weave. Speciality wig shops can offer realistic looking synthetic materials.

   However, as many a man who has shamefully lost his toupee to a strong gust of wind, hairpieces are artificial, may look unnatural, and may simply fall off at the worst of times.

b. **Hair restoration:** Hair transplantation is a permanent form of hair replacement. Anyone who has suffered permanent hair loss may be a candidate for hair transplantation.

   The surgical transplanting of hair follicles is a remarkably simple outpatient procedure. The procedure of hair transplantation involves moving some hair-bearing portions (donor sites) of the head (usually the horse-shoe-shaped area at the very back of the head), to bald or thinning portions, (recipient sites) and/or removing bald skin.

c. **A full head of hair:** With proper techniques, and solutions, hair loss can be minimized. If you suffer from hair loss, invest the time and research treatment options and weigh the benefits of replacing lost or thinning hair.

   After all, a full head of hair not only influences the way others perceive you professionally and personally, but can influence the way you view yourself.

Questions

INTRODUCTION

a. Why do many women now have blocked fallopian tubes?
b. Define fallopian tube.
c. Explain what happens, when a fallopian tube is blocked?
d. Name four types of blocked fallopian tubes?
e. Name seven causes of blocked fallopian tube?
f. What are the symptoms of blocked fallopian tube?
g. What is fibroid?
h. What is the medical name for fibroid?
i. Which category of women does fibroid affects?
j. State four complications that uterine fibroid may lead to?
k. What are the treatment for fibroid?
l. What are the seven sympyoms of uterine ffibroid?
m. Suggest a cure for fibroid?
n. Where is fibroid found in woman's body

SICKNESS IS A SPIRIT

a. What does mark 9:25, Luke 13:11-112, James 4:7, and Mark 5:8-1 says about sickness?
b. Is sickness really a spirit? Discuss

LAUGH YOUR WAY TO GOOD HEALTH

    a. What do you really learn from all the jokes?

    b. What does alcohol eventually does to an organ in the body?

ARTHRITIS

    a. What is arthritis? Discuss.

    b. Name three types of arthritis?

    c. Enumerate, and discuss the types of treatment for arthritis?

    d. Name the medications that ca n be given to arthritis patients?

    e. What is heat theraphy?

    f. What is cold theraphy?

    g. Discuss hydrotheraphy, mobilization therapies, and relaxation therapies?

    h. Name the assistive devices, that are used to support weak joints? What will happen if such devicee does not fit properly to the patient?

    i. Is surgery required to repair joint damage aafter trauma? Discuss.

    j. Naame the drugs that can be used to treat arthritis?

    k. Discuss massage, acupuncture, the Alexander technique, aromatherapht, chiropractic, osteopathy, and reflexology?

HOW COUPLE CAN COPE WITH INFERTILITY.

    a. Discuss six ways couples can cope with infertility?

    b. Should infertile couples take part in support groups?

    c. What is vagina discharge?

    d. What are the causes of vaginal discharge?

    e. Do men have sexual problems? Discuss.

    f. What is annovulation?

    g. What causes blocked fallopian tube in some women? Suggest a solution to it.

    h. What can antibodies in a woman does to the male sperm?

    i. Name two drugs that can be used, if hormone is the cause of infertility?

j. How can women cope with toilet disease discharge?
k. What does abnormalities in discharge indicate in a woman?
l. Yeast, candida, albicans cause itching in the tropical region, discuss?
m. Name two drugs that can be used to treat candida albican? Name other two solutions to vaginal itching outside orthodox medicine?
n. What is bacteria vaginosis?
o. What is trichomonas? Discuss.
p. What is gardenalia? Is laboratory test necessary in treating it?
q. State two general mode of preventing gardenalia, and discuss?

FOOD POISONING

a. What is food poisoning?
b. Enumerate, and discuss seven standard guidelines for people going for late dinner?
c. Enumerate, and discuss eight standard guidelines for dinner host?
d. How can food poisoning be managed? Name the three drugs that can be used to manage it?
e. "Beware, food poisoning is real" Discuss.
f. Enumerate the illness that can accompany food poisoning?
g. Discuss two ways that food poisoning organisms can enter the body?
h. What are the precautionary measures to take in preventing food poisoning?
i. State ten tips on preventing food poisoning?

LEMON GRASS

a. What is lemon grass? Discuss it's anti-cancer properties.
b. What can lemon grass be used for?
c. State three principal constituents of lemon grass?

BITTER LEAF

a. State the World Health Organisation definition of childlessness?
b. State the four causes of infertility in men and women?
c. Does bitter leaves combined with Russian peniciline vegetable cure infertility related diseases? Discuss.

PALM OIL

a. What is the characteristic of palm oil?
b. Whaat vitamin does it contain?
c. What will deficiency of this vitamin leads to?
d. What are carotenoids/ Name the six carotenoids you know?
e. What does beta-carotene prevents, and how?
f. State the other sources of vitamin A?
g. Enumerate twenty six food that contains significant amount of vitamin A?
h. Enumerate twenty nine herbs that contains significant amount of vitamin A?
i. State three drugs that interfere with vitamin A?
j. State the daily dose of vitamin A allowed a pregnant woman?

HONEY

a. Honey is a valuable food supplement? Discuss.
b. What are the properties of pure honey?
c. What are the benefits of honey?
d. What are the uses of honey?
e. How can pure honey be identified?
f. How is honey marketed internationally?

FRUITS THAT ENHANCE YOUR SKIN

a. State seven fruits that are beneficial to the skin?
b. What will these fruits give the body?
c. What six advise can be recommended to enhance the skin?

CANCER

a. What is cancer?
b. State the six most common cancer tumors?
c. Who is an oncologist?
d. How can six types of cancer be diagnosed?
e. State the new test measure to use in detecting breast cancer?
f. Red wine do cut the risk of ovarian cancer. Discuss.
g. What does drinking wine does to a woman's body?
h. What is personal breast screening?

BREAST CANCER

a. What is a breast, and it's functions?
b. What is breast cancer?
c. What does it means, if a breast lump is benign, or malignant?
d. State two risk factors that initiate or facilitate the cancerous process?
e. What are the intrinsic factors?
f. What are the extrinsic factors?
g. What are the six signs of breast cancer?
h. List seven types of breast examination?
i. State five factors that can be controlled in order to prevent breast cancer?
j. State five treatments of breast cancer?
k. State five long term or non reversible side effects of breast cancer?
l. State four ways that can be used to manage the side effect of breast cancer?
m. Tate five contents of complementary theraphy?
n. Discuss two steps necessary in discovering breast cancer?

QUICK HEALING STRATEGIES FOR ULCER

a. Discuss the quick healing strategies of ulcer?
b. Name the acid that cause ulcer in the body?
c. What are the common signs and symptoms of ulcer?
d. How can ulcer be treated?

e. State the two types of surgeries for ulcer patients?
f. What can untreated ulcer cause over a long period?
g. What are the doctors advise to ulcer patients?
h. Discuss the eleven important fast healing strategies for ulcer?

EFFECTIVE DIABETES TREATMENTS FOR PATIENTS

a. What are the three primary causes of diabetes?
b. Name the hormone produced, and it's source in the body? Explain the function of insulin?
c. Name the abdominal fat protein that mess up the mechanism of insulin as a key?
d. What three organs can diabetes damage?
e. What three effects does insulin resistance cause to the body?
f. What is the solution in preventing diabetes?
g. Name the drug that can be use in treating diabetic patients?
h. Does diabetes occurs in children? Discuss.
i. State seven do's in controlling diabetes?
j. What is the name of herbs used in curing diabetes?
k. What four things should people with diabetes do?

STAPHYLOCCOCUS

a. Define staphylococcus? Explain.
b. What three effects can staphylococcus have on hormones?
c. How many species of staphylococcus identified by medical experts?
d. Name four types of staphylococcus, and the areas of human body they affects, and effects?
e. State seven organs and parts of the body that staphylococcus affects, and effects?

HYPERTENSION RISKS

a. What are the things that can cause one's risk of hypertension?
b. Discuss hypertension risks?

LIFE SAVING NEWS ABOUT STROKE

   a. What are the five symptoms of stroke?

AROMATHERAPY RELIEVES PAINS

   a. What does aromatherapy does to human body?
   b. What are the two uses of aromatherapy?
   c. What six things should one do to use aromatherapy for pain relaxation, and rejuvenation?

PROSTATE ENLARGEMENT

   a. What is prostate enlargement?
   b. What eleven symptoms occurs, when an enlarge prostate gland exerts pressure on the urethra?

EFFECTIVE WAYS TO AVOID MOUTH ODOUR

   a. What are the causes of bad breath?
   b. Name he chemical compounds emitted by the mouth of a person with mouth odours?
   c. What are the twelve factors that can lead to mouth odour?
   d. State seven self help antidotes to mouth odour?
   e. How can cancer of the mouth, and throat be prevented?
   f. What causes oral cancer?
   g. What are the importance of early detection of oral cancer?
   h. What two factors increase the risk of lip cancer?
   i. Regular dental check-up's important. Discuss.

BACTERIA WORSEN ASTHMA IN KIDS

   a. Name the bacteria that is responsible for triggering asthma attacks in children?
   b. State two respiratory infections?

PLEASE, STOP THE POLIO INFECTION IN CHILDREN.

a. What does polio cause in children?
b. What is a virus?
c. What is the mode of transmission of polio in children? State the age of infectons?
d. How many drops of polio vaccines are needed, over what period to escape from the danger posed by polio?
e. State two things that oral polio vaccines does to the children's body?
f. Why is immunization significant in children?
g. Explain the factors that pose serious challenges to polio eradication?

WHAT TO KNOW ABOUT PERIODS OR MENSTRUATIONS.

a. Explain the process of menstruation?
b. State four general guides of menstrual blood?
c. What is menopause?
d. At what age ranges can menopause occur?
e. Can food supplements cub the stress of menopause? Explain
f. Are there some things a lady may lose at menopause, apart from her menses?
g. What happens when al hormones are no longer in a woman's body due to menopause?
h. Discuss hot flashes experienced by menopausal women?
i. What advise can be given to menopausal women?
j. What is menopause?
k. What are the causes of menopause?
l. State three complications of menopause?
m. What factors affects the beginning of menopause in women?
n. Explain what happens when a woman experience menopause?
o. Can a woman be pregnant after menopause? Explain.
p. What is the name of a new contraceptive use to avoid conception in women?
q. What is it's period of effectiveness, and state the percentage of it's effectiveness?

DO YOU KNOW THAT SNORING CAN LEAD TO PREMATURE DEATH?

a. What effects can snoring pose to human health, and the social life of a person, that snores?
b. Site an example of what snoring had caused in a marital relationship?
c. What is snoring?
d. Why do people snore?
e. Sleep and relaxation goes hand in hand. Explain.
f. What health attacks can snoring cause?
g. Snoring can be inherited. Explain?
h. What effect does smoking, and exposure to second-hand smoke cause?
i. State and explain the seven self-help tips to prevent or alleviate snoring?

BLEACHING OF THE SKIN

a. Is bleaching dangerous? Explain.
b. What is bleaching of the skin? Explain.
c. Describe skin?
d. What are the causes of bleaching skin?
e. Who started bleaching, and in what country, and why?

STOPPING HAIR LOSS

a. What are the available options for men that suffers hair loss?
b. Name the two drugs used in treating hair loss?
c. Why do bald men wear wigs, toupes or weave?
d. Explain the process of hair transplantation?
e. What effects can a full head hair cause?